Introduction to Hospital Management

Introduction to Hospital Management

C. Charles

ANMOL PUBLICATIONS PVT. LTD.
NEW DELHI - 110 002 (INDIA)

ANMOL PUBLICATIONS PVT. LTD.
H.O.: 4374/4B, Ansari Road, Darya Ganj
New Delhi-110 002 (India)
Ph.: 23278000, 23261597
B.O.: 1015, Ist Main Road, BSK IIIrd Stage
IIIrd Phase, IIIrd Block
Bangalore - 560 085 (Karnataka)
Ph: 080-41723429, Tel/Fax: 080-2672 3604
Visit us at: www.anmolpublications.com

Introduction to Hospital Management

First Published, 2008

ISBN 978-81-261-3283-6

PRINTED IN INDIA

Printed at Mehra Offset Press, Delhi.

Contents

	Preface	*vii*
1.	Introduction to Hospital Management	1
2.	List of Hospital Departments	75
3.	Select List of Hospitals in India	77
4.	Select List of Hospitals Worldwide	84
5.	Select List of Diseases	170
	Bibliography	325
	Index	327

Preface

Hospital represents any institution duly licensed, certified, and operated as a hospital. In no event should the term "Hospital" include a convalescent facility, nursing home, or any institution or part thereof which is used principally as a convalescence facility, rest facility, nursing facility, or facility for the aged. Hospital case management is a collaborative process that assesses, plans, implements, coordinates, monitors and evaluates the options and services required to meet an individual's health needs, using communication and available resources to promote quality, cost-effective outcomes in the hospital environment. A hospital case manager coordinates the clinical goals with the patient's goals and manages the financial and quality outcomes of the care provided. With appropriate training, education and direction, hospital case managers can use their skills to affect a balanced clinical and financial outcome. Health is the state of complete physical, mental, and social well-being and not merely the absence of disease or infirmity. It is recognized, however, that health has many dimensions (anatomical, physiological, and mental) and is largely culturally defined. The relative importance of various disabilities will differ depending upon the cultural milieu and the role of the affected individual in that culture. Most attempts at measurement have been assessed in terms or morbidity and mortality.

Health care implies care, services, and supplies related to the health of an individual. Health care includes preventive, diagnostic, therapeutic, rehabilitative, maintenance, or palliative care, and counseling, among other services.

Healthcare also includes the sale and dispensing of prescription drugs or devices Health administration focuses on community organization and community health, health systems research, public health legislations, urban health, health policy formulation and implementation, financing of health services, management of national health programs and so on, hospital management aims at social services in hospitals, financial management organization and administration of clinical/support services, legal frame work of hospitals, hospital planning, quality assurance, marketing management, strategic management and information management.

This publication entitled "Introduction to Hospital Management" is published specifically to clarify the business, medical and operational aspects of healthcare management in the modern age. The focus lies on key issues, including innovative medical technologies, patient care and medical treatments. Hospital Management as a career has come to the forefront in the sphere of professions only recently. However, a Hospital Manager's job would be interesting and replete with responsibilities all at once. In the days gone by, a very senior doctor was generally assigned the role of a hospital manager. But in this era of specialization, the term hospital has undergone manifold changes and many categories have been chalked out. So, now you have ordinary hospitals, specialty hospitals and even super specialty hospitals depending upon the kinds of services they render to the public and the number of people they cater to, on an average. In earlier times many ordinary people dreaded to go to hospitals, fearing that it was a death trap, from where they would never return. That myth has now been dispelled. Nowadays hospitals are considered, and indeed prove to be, utterly comfortable nay luxurious, where the patients in various stages of diseases can enjoy privacy and peace of mind. As a natural consequence, several courses and training programmes have been evolved to churn out professional hospital mangers and give the veteran doctors a breathing space. Such individuals are by far exceedingly well -equipped to face the growing challenges and cater to the specific requirements of modern day hospitals.

This publication entitled "Introduction to Hospital Management" can be used as a reference book for current opinion and the latest developments in the field of hospital administration and management, such as, cardiovascular equipment and devices; cleaning and disinfections management; communications and telemedicine; critical care; diagnostics and analysis; facilities management; furniture and fittings; healthcare courses, training and events; healthcare informatics; hospital security systems; implants and fixation devices; laboratory equipment; medical and surgical disposables; medical clothing; medical imaging and diagnostics; patient monitoring; pharmaceuticals and medicines; rehabilitation and mobility; respiratory care and anesthesiology; sterilization; surgical and electro-surgical equipment; and wound-care and dressings.

—Editor

1

Introduction to Hospital Management

HOSPITAL SYSTEMS

The Need for Reform

Hospital systems are integral parts of health care delivery . Hospitals are, in varying degrees, vital resources for patient care, health manpower development and research. Hospital care is also the most expensive component of health care. With the high cost of hospital construction and enormous operating costs, the peso value of its material resources and the size of its staff, it can easily gobble up a large portion of the national health budget and impoverish the rest of the health services.

There are several areas in the present set-up of government hospitals that need reforms. Foremost of these are the provincial and district hospitals, which were devolved with the noble intention of bringing primary, secondary and even tertiary hospital services nearer to the people. These hospitals were intended to be managed by the provincial governments, which were more aware of the health needs of the locality. However, implementation problems did not attain the noble intention of devolution of health services leading to the deterioration of these facilities.

This pathetic predicament can be demonstrated in a cycle of inadequacy and aggravation. The lack of even the primary and secondary hospital services in the provincial and district hospitals forced the patients to seek hospital care in the regional and national hospitals which were retained by the national government. The expected result of congestion in these regional and national hospitals is now apparent. Such congestion aggravated the chronic understaffing of these regional and national hospitals affecting the quality of health services. The irrational delivery of primary and secondary hospital services in these supposedly tertiary level and referral hospitals further lead to cost-inefficiency and bigger share in the DOH budget.

More than 50 percent of the annual DOH budget goes to hospital services. Moreover, with the deterioration of hospital services in the provincial and district hospitals, the congestion of tertiary level regional and national hospitals, and the irrational delivery of hospital services paralyzed the promotive and preventive aspects of health care in these facilities.

The inadequacies in the government hospital system is further aggravated by inadequate private-public hospital networking and patient referral system.

Objectives

- In sync with local health system reforms, upgrade the provincial and district hospitals to strengthen the delivery of promotive and preventive health services and primary, secondary and, in selected provincial hospitals, even tertiary curative services.
- Upgrade the regional and national hospitals to strengthen capability for tertiary and specialized end-referral hospital services, training and research and, at the same time strengthen promotive and preventive health services.
- In parallel with the expansion of health insurance

coverage, convert regional and national hospitals into fiscally autonomous facilities and, eventually, into financially viable government corporations.

— As financially stable government corporations, reduce the dependence of these hospitals on direct public subsidies and, eventually, free-up government resources for other priorities (like public health programmes and local health systems development).

— Strengthen government and private hospital networking and patient referral systems and, eventually, work towards the development of the Philippine Hospital System.

Goal

To convert government hospitals into fiscally autonomous entities and develop the Philippine Hospital System with the private sector.

Reform Strategies

Parallel and Rational Revitalisation of Provincial and District Hospitals Together with the Regional and National Hospitals

The first strategic approach is the revitalisation of the provincial and district hospitals. Parallel to this is the continuous upgrading of the regional and national hospitals and the establishment of regional specialty centers. All these are envisioned in the Philippine Hospital Development Plan.

In the area-based hospital development plans, the rationalized upgrading of provincial, cityand district hospitals, including the military hospitals under the Department of National Defense,are included. These area-based plans will be presented to the local government executives for their support and commitment to be formalized through a Memorandum of Agreement. Later, private hospitals, as part of the Philippine Hospital Systems, will be included in these plans. The area based hospital development plans will be the major basis for the public investment plan of the hospitals.

The revitalisation of the provincial and district hospitals will need tremendous human resource development for which the staff of the regional and national hospitals and the DOH central office will serve as trainers and resource persons. Complementary with the human resource development will be the rationalized service capability upgrading through infrastructure (including solid waste and waste-water treatment facilities), equipment, supplies and information systems development.

The Philippine Hospital Development Plan intends to upgrade the regional and national hospitals into state-of-the-art tertiary level hospitals with capability for even the highly specialized curative and rehabilitative services. In addition, regional specialty centers such as heart-lung-kidney centers, pediatric centers, oncology centers, toxicology centers, among others, will be established in strategic medical centers in Mindanao, Visayas and Luzon.

At the upper end of the referral system are the national centers for specialized health services. These centers are the existing specialty centers (Philippine Heart Center, National Kidney and Transplant Institute, Philippine Children's Medical Center, and Lung Center of the Philippines), and the proposed neuroscience center, hematology center and blood transfusion center. These specialized centers will compose the Philippine Centers for Specialized Health Care.

The critical upgrading of capacities of the provincial and districts hospitals must be in parallel with the upgrading of national and regional hospitals. The parallel upgrading is necessary to prevent congestion of tertiary care facilities with primary care patients. It is also necessary to prevent displacement of true indigent patients when the regional and national hospitals unload patients to give way to increased number of pay and private rooms as they become fiscally autonomous and financially viable. This strategy shall be linked with the goal of universal coverage under the National Health Insurance Programme.

Guided and Phased-in Conversion of Regional and National Hospitals into Government Corporations or Other Appropriate Government Institutions

The third strategic approach is a guided and phased in conversion of these regional and national hospitals into government corporations based on the current and projected financial picture. At present national hospitals are experiencing a very high occupancy rate ranging from 100 to 120 percent of authorized bed capacity. This overutilized medical facilities can be categorized financially into three groups:

Group I: Selected Metro Manila medical centers with 95 percent indigent patients and negative budget.

Group II: Regional hospitals and medical centers with high percentage of indigent patients with no provincial and district hospitals to unload to but with high potential for income generating hospital services.

Group III: National hospitals with a reasonable number of private rooms and pay wards with high potential for increased income-generation.

Based on the current financial picture of hospitals, the conversion into government corporations will most logically be phased-in. Those in group 1 must first become financially stable then viable. This will need a strong political will and sound financial management to turn around its negative finances to financially viable undertaking. Those in group

2 are more likely to become financially stable and viable but will need more time to be converted to government corporations. Those in group 3 are the potential candidates for conversion into government corporations within the short-term period.

Expansion of Hospital Financing Systems of the Regional and National Hospitals

The second strategic approach is the expansion of hospital financing systems in tandem with the continuous upgrading of the regional and national hospitals into income-generating and financially viable health facilities complementing the private sector. Government hospitals should be allowed to collect, retain and allocate revenue from socialized user fees and other forms of revenue-generating activities.

The following mechanisms to expand the sources for hospital financing should be included:

(a) Revenue enhancement through increased number of pay wards, private rooms, and doctors' OPD clinics, and expanded hospital services for ambulatory surgical care and domiciliary care.

(b) Review and implement the appropriate hospital fees and charges.

(c) Stricter collection of hospital service fees through voucher system and other effective means.

(d) More efficient utilisation of the hospital income from the income-generating areas (laboratory, x-ray, delivery room, operating room, etc.). This can be done by decreasing the turn-around time for the return of hospital income from the Bureau of Treasury to the Department of Budget and Management and back to the DOH. Also, the possibility of making hospital income as revolving funds can be explored.

(e) Expand the sources of hospital revolving funds such

as proceeds from sale of drugs and medicines. Hospital pharmacies need to be upgraded and competitive to increase their income from the paying public. This endeavor is being undertaken through the "DOH Botika" project.

(f) Expand the health insurance coverage (potential hospital patients) and the package of hospital services to be reimbursed by the health insurance system.

Given all these possible sources of revenue enhancement and with financial analysts and health economists assisting the hospital managers, tremendous improvement in hospital financing systems is expected.

As the regional and national hospitals become more financially sustained from their own income, dependence on direct government subsidies can eventually be reduced to free-up more money for other DOH priorities like public health programmes. At present, the annual budget from the national government per hospital is tremendously inadequate compared to the supposed budget derived from the recommended case-mixed or activity-based budgeting. With this predicament, the hospitals are already under-budgeted and the present hospital income generated is still low to compensate for the under-budgeting. If government subsidy will be reduced, hospital managers fear that the income will not be sufficient to maintain expenses for efficient hospital operations and quality patient care. Toaddress this fear, a few remedial measures are proposed:

(a) Set the target percentage for the reduction of public subsidy to government hospitals, giving the hospital management more options for recovery of the reduced amount from other sources, (i.e., increased hospital income, external funding sources, etc.) provided the present capacities of the hospitals are upgraded.

(b) Establish mechanisms for continued public subsidy through a multi-year budgeting to give the hospital management a clear picture of how much and when subsidies come for a proactive budget planning and financial management. c. Diversify and mobilize other fund sources, both from government or external sources through projects, grants-in-aid, etc.

Integration of Appropriate and Priority Public Health Programmes into Hospital Services

The integration of public health programmes within hospital services will require additional staff within the hospital like health educators and public health specialists. Public Health Units shall be established as the main venue for the provision of promotive and preventive health services within the hospitals. Public health personnel may also be tapped to augment the present hospital staff in some aspects of curative care. This will partly answer the chronic hospital problem of under-staffing.

Expansion of the Existing Government Hospital Networking and Patient Referral System to Include Private Hospitals and Form the Philippine Hospital System

The fourth strategic approach consist of strengthening government and private hospital networking and patient referral and, eventually, the formation of the Philippine Hospital System. It is envisioned that the same set of standards will govern all hospitals inclusive of the private and the government sector. One concrete example is the Integrated Hospital Information System under the Hospital Epidemiology Programme where all government and private hospitals will have the same software. Through the Philippine Hospital System, indigent patients can avail of private hospital services through subsidy from the DOH indigency funds and through the national health insurance programme. Further, through the same system, indigent patients can avail of specialized diagnostic and therapeutic services that are available only in selected private hospitals. Training programmes in private hospitals can also be accessed by government hospital personnel and vice versa.

For private hospitals, the Philippine Hospital System will open opportunities for participation in government health programmes, particularly foreign-assisted projects made available to government hospitals. Many other advantages and opportunities can be seen as the Philippine Hospital System materializes.

Policy Action Needed

Grant Fiscal Autonomy or Corporate Status to Government Hospitals

Include as special provision in the General Appropriations Act the granting of fiscal autonomy to government hospitals by allowing them to manage their income and retain this income as revolving funds to augment their current budgetary allocation. This will eventually reduce their dependence on yearly government subsidy and free-up resources for other health priorities. Financially viable government hospitals should be converted into government corporations with the primary objective of maintaining sustainability of operations rather than profit, thereby retaining their social responsibilities.

Moratorium on All Hospital Re-nationalisation Efforts

There is a need for moratorium on all hospital renationalisation efforts. Provision of direct health services, particularly, primary and secondary hospital care, even some tertiary health care should remain as the responsibility of the local government units.

Enhance Health Facility Development

Under the Philippine Hospital Development Plan,

national government hospitals will be strengthened in order to cope up with the ever-increasing demand for hospital services brought about by population aging and life expectancy increases. The same scheme shall also address the decline in service capability of provincial and district hospitals which had been devolved pursuant to the passage of the Local Government Code.

Related to this plan, a bill known as "The National Health Facilities Enhancement Act," was filed in the Senate. The bill provides for a National Health Facilities Fund where both government and private hospitals can financially benefit. If passed into law, The National Health Facilities Enhancement Act together with the Philippine Hospital Development Plan can rejuvenate the ailing hospital system of the country.

Organisational Changes Needed

Convert Government Hospitals into Government Corporations

The conversion of government hospitals, particularly the regional and national hospitals, into government corporations will entail simultaneous studies on the legal basis, financial viability, and technical capability of candidate hospitals. Hospital corporate boards need to be organised with the Regional Health Directors and Local Health Executives, among others, as part of the membership. Systems and processes for policy and decision making and financial management need to be developed along corporate set-up.

Simultaneously with the organisational change in government hospitals, an office within the health operations cluster at the DOH Central Office need to be organised to provide the following functions:

(a) Formulate policies and guidelines on the operations

and management of hospitals and other health facilities;

(b) Formulate a national plan for the development and equitable distribution of hospitals and other health facilities;

(c) Institute hospital reforms towards fiscal autonomy and corporatisation;

(d) Provide technical assistance in financing hospitals and other health facilities; and

(e) Provide technical support in the development of health facility resources (e.g., human resources, infrastructure, equipment, etc.).

(f) Develop networking and coordination mechanisms for national and local as well as government and private hospitals and health facilities.

Institutionalize Financial and Procurement Systems

Hospital fiscal and management autonomy will entail improvement in hospital systems and subsystems particularly in financial management and procurement. This will require amendment of certain existing administrative rules and regulations. However, in most areas, improvement in the implementation of accounting, bidding procedures and sound supply management will lead to maximum utilisation and prioritisation of hospital resources.

Rationalize Development, Production, Distribution and Utilisation of Health Human Resources

Addressing the present complex problems in health human resources will entail coordination of current efforts to equitably distribute much needed health professionals and augment hospital staffing in accordance to standards and diagnosis-related groupings. Present efforts include coordination with Specialty Societies, residency dispersal, consortium of hospitals for sharing of consultants and specialists, incentives for doctors assigned to difficult-to-reach areas. The endgoal for these efforts is to synchronize health human resource development with the service capability upgrading under the Philippine Hospital Development Plan.

Public Investments Needed

Upgrade Critical Capacities in Government Hospitals

Investments for government hospital reforms will be directed towards rationalized upgrading of hospitals (both DOH- and LGU-operated hospitals), including repair and upgrading of physical plant, provision of equipment, human resource development, and some operating costs. This will involve 276 hospitals – 156 core district hospitals, 78 provincial hospitals, 20 medical centers, 11 regional hospitals, 6 special hospitals, and 2 research hospitals and at least 12 Metro Manila City Hospitals.

Improving the critical capacities of these government hospitals is primarily intended to make them more competitive and responsive to the health needs of their clientele. This will enable government hospitals to effectively exercise fiscal autonomy and, eventually, facilitate their conversion to government corporations without compromising their social responsibilities.

Enhance Government Hospital Revenue Towards Fiscal Autonomy and Conversion to Government Corporations

Mechanisms for enhancing revenue sources for government hospitals should be instituted. Government hospitals should be allowed to collect, retain and allocate revenue from their own income and convert them, initially, into fiscally autonomous facilities. Once financial viability is established, these hospitals should be converted into government corporations.

Expand Hospital Networking and Patient Re-ferral System

Investment is necessary to expand networking and patient referral system between the national and local health facilities and between the government and private sectors. Hospital Information Systems need to be developed and linked from one facility to another and with the national health insurance programme. Sharing of expertise, facilities and other resources between national and local health facilities and between government and private health facilities should be tapped. A strong link among facilities would expedite the formation of the Philippine Hospital System.

Time Table for Major Reform Activities

Strategy	*Years 1–2*	*Years 3–51.*
1. Upgrade critical capacities of government hospitals	— Upgrade selected hospitals (those that are ready for fiscal autononomy or corporatisation)	— Upgrade DOH and LGUhospitals in Mindanao
	— Upgrade DOH and LGU hospitals in Luzon and Metro Manila	— Upgrade DOH and LGU hospitals in the Visayas
2. Provide fiscal autonomy or corporate set-up	— Convert Group 3 hospitals into corporate entities	— Convert Group 2 hospitals into corporate entities
	— Convert Group 2 hospitals into fiscally autonomous facilities	— Convert Group 1 hospitals into fiscally autonomous facilities
3. Strengthen government and private hospital net-working	— Expand hospital networkingand referral systems among DOH and LGU hospitals	— Expand government andprivate hospital networking
	— Develop linkages with private hospitals	— Strengthen the Philippine Hospital System
4. Expand hospital finaning	— Enhance revenues	— Create hospital management board as interim tocorporate board
	— Retain and utilize income	— Expand insurance coverage
5. Integrate priority public health programmes into hospital services	— Establish public health unitsin hospitals	— Recovery from intensive care
	— Implement DOTS and otherpublic health programmes	

RECOVERY FROM INTENSIVE CARE

Studies of outcome after intensive care suggest that death rates do not return to normal until 2-4 years after admission.Although some questionnaire studies have reported on morbidity,little published work exists on detailed clinical recovery orlonger term residual effects of critical illness. The recoveryprocess may present serious physical, psychological, and socialproblems for both patients and their families, and these may lastfor months or years. Although patients who have been in intensivecare have often been extremely ill, been at high risk of death,and received care costing tens of thousands of pounds, detailedfollow up and targeted support are still rare.

Examples of Physical Disorders After Intensive Care

— Recovering organ failure (lung, kidney, liver, etc)

— Severe muscle wasting and weakness including reduced cough power, pharyngeal weakness

— Joint stiffness

— Numbness, paraesthesia (peripheral neuropathy)

— Taste changes resulting in favourite foods being unpalatable

— Disturbances to sleep rhythm

— Cardiac and circulatory decompensation:
Postural hypotension

— Reduced pulmonary reserve:
Breathlessness on mild exertion

— Iatrogenic:
Tracheal stenosis (for example, from repeated intubations) Nerve palsies (needle injuries) Scarring (needle and drain sites)

The commonest physical problem reported by intensive care patients is severe weakness and fatigue. Patients in intensive carecan lose about 2% of muscle mass a day during their illness owingto a combination of primary muscle catabolism and atrophy secondaryto neuropathic degeneration. They may lose over half their musclemass, resulting in severe physical disability. Rebuilding suchmuscle losses can take over a year. Initially, patients may beso weak that they struggle to feed themselves, their cough poweris greatly reduced, and they may have poor control of their swallowingand upper airways with a risk of aspiration. The nursing burdencan be large. If patients can stand they are in danger of falling.This is often compounded by postural hypotension, which may reflectautonomic disturbances

On discharge from intensive care patients may seem completely oriented and to understand the information they are given abouttheir illness. Yet when questioned a few days later, many havelittle or no memory of their stay in intensive care or can rememberonly pain, suctioning, or lack of sleep. The only memories ofsome patients are nightmares, often of a persecutory nature inwhich they are subjected to torture, or paranoid delusions. These nightmares and delusions may be attributed to the illness, theuse of opiate and sedative drugs, the unnatural environment ofintensive care with its lack of a proper day and night, and toconstant noise. Patients nursed in an intensive care unit withoutwindows have even more unpleasant memories than those nursed ina unit with large windows.

Taste changes and difficulties in feeding themselves may further compromise patients' nutritional state

The difficulty some patients have in accepting that the events in their dreams were not real is often not appreciated. Inaddition, patients are reluctant to tell ward staff about theirnightmares for fear of being considered mad. However, confrontation,through discussion, of such problems allows patients to buildup a coherent story rather than chaotic, intrusive memories andso put the experience behind them. The incidence of post-traumaticstress disorder is high after intensive care, and it is more commonin patients who recall frightening adverseexperiences.

Patient's View

A 42 year old woman with acute pancreatitis required a 40 day stay in intensive care. She had been ill in hospital for several weeks before transfer. When she went home she found she had lost 2 months from her memory the time in intensive care and in the ward before that. She worried about what had happened to her and why she could not remember.

She learnt about her illness and why she could not remember at the follow up clinic. She was relieved that there was nothing wrong with her mind and that it is common not to be able to remember.

When patients first see themselves in the mirror they may not recognise their face because of severe weight loss. With nomemory of their illness, patients have no explanation for thisfrightening confrontation, and they may also find it difficultto appreciate why they feel so awful. For example, they may onlyremember coming in for elective surgery and waking up on the ward,seemingly the next morning, and be left thinking "why have I lostall this weight, why am I soweak?"

Discharge to the Ward

Patients on mechanical ventilation are usually discharged from the intensive care unit to the ward when they can breathe unaided.However, several physical problems may still remain. Althoughthese may not be serious enough to keep the patient in intensivecare, if left untreated they could lead to readmission. Intensivecare staff should therefore follow patients' progress on the wardfor a few days to monitor recovery of multisystem disease andassure good continuity of care.

Discharge Home

It is often when patients go home that they realise how debilitated they are; commonly, they cannot climb stairs. Relativestake on the care of the patients and, for example, report sleeplessnessbecause of worry about whether the patient is still breathing.Relatives often report that patients are hard to live with becauseof irritability and impatience with the slowness of theirrecovery.

> **Relative's View**
>
> After John's wife had been in intensive care he felt that it was better that she didn't know about her illness and so wouldn't discuss it. He had been very upset and wanted to protect her. He could not bring himself to return to hospital, even to accompany his wife to outpatient clinics. His wife was initially upset by this behaviour. However, once she had been told how ill she had been she understood how much stress John had been under and his subsequent behaviour.

Many healthcare professionals believe that it is better for patients not to remember their intensive care stay. This meansthat patients are unable to explain why they feel so debilitated.Although the family may try to explain, the lack of a concretememory makes it difficult for patients to realise just how illthey have been and just how long it will take them to recover.Patients consequently have unrealistic expectations of recoveryand think in terms of weeks instead of months, if notyears.

Except for very elderly and some trauma and neurological patients, most intensive care patients will not receive any physiotherapyonce they are able to walk unaided in hospital. However, muscleloss and peripheral neuropathies may affect their balance, andthey have poor ability to right themselves. Walking unaided outsidein icy conditions or in a wind is potentially dangerous and frighteningfor the patient. In addition, minor physical problems such ashair loss, skin dryness, or fingernail ridges, which often occurafter critical illness can be particularly distressing becauseof the lack of an adequate explanation during the dischargeprocess.

Two Months to One Year

Physical problems related to muscle weakness are still common 2 months after intensive care and can still be seen at 6 months.These problems often affect self care activities such as climbingstairs, getting out of the bath, turning off taps, driving a car,and returning to work. Fear of falling and being unable to getup again is common.

Psychological Disorders

- Depression:
  Anger and conflict with the family
- Anxiety:
  Are they going to get back to normal?
  Panic attacks
  Fear of dying
- Guilt
- Recurrent nightmares
- Post traumatic stress disorder

Actual Examples of Problems Reported by Patients

"I get panicky if I go out alone in case I am taken ill"

"I get very angry with my family. They keep fussing when I try to do things for myself"

"I feel very angry with myself for not being back to normal by now"

"I've tried to help by doing the washing up but I keep dropping the crockery"

"When I first went home I climbed the stairs on my hands and knees and came down on my bottom"

"I don't want to go to sleep because I keep dreaming that I'm back in ICU"

> "My whole time in ICU I dreamt I had been kidnapped and locked in the boot of a car"
>
> "I feel very guilty when I think about what my family has been through"

The prolonged recovery period leads to several problems, and intensive care survivors experience considerable levels of depressionand anxiety. Patients often avoid company and show less affectionto their partners. In one study 45% of patients questioned at6 months reported going out less often, 41% took part in fewersocial activities, and a quarter reported being irritable withtheirrelatives.

Coupled to this social isolation is a dependence on others to make decisions and a tendency towards being obstinate. Patientsalso report feeling overwhelmed in crowded places or being afraidto go out alone. Some patients describe full blown panic attacks,although they may not necessarily recognise them as such. Thelonger panic attacks are left untreated, the more refractory theyare likely to be. Long term treatment is needed by 36-40% of peoplewith panic attacks presenting forhelp.

Patients understandably feel that the recovery phase of their critical illness is the most stressful period as they have tocome to terms with how ill and close to death they have been.The presence of social support increases tolerance to stressfulsituations and has, in general, a beneficial effect on health.Social isolation, however, seems to act as a source of chronicstress. Much of the impact caused by life events may be the resultof the profound changes they produce in social relationships.

Guide to Care after Hospital Discharge

Integration of physical and psychological care is clearly in the best interest of these patients. What issues need to be addressedwhen planning for hospital discharge for intensive care patients?A partnership is needed between the patient's general practitioner,ward doctor, and intensive care doctor. Clear information aboutthe illness should be provided to patients, their families, andtheir general practitioners. Patients need to be given some ideaabout how long it will take them to recover. Both patients andtheir families should be given the opportunity to be debriefedabout the illness, the time in intensive care, and what it means,preferably by staff who were involved in the patients' care. Debriefingshould tackle not only the reasons for admission to intensivecare and events while they were there but also any distorted memoriespatients may have. For many patients, simply knowing that nightmaresand paranoid delusions are normal after critical illness is sufficientfor them to put the memories in context.

Guide for Care after Discharge

— Initial review by intensive care staff to ensure medical and nursing handover is thorough, seamless, and continuous

— Early explanation of illness to patient, preferably with a relative present to ensure uniformity of experience

— Advice to patients on problems and information on the time scale of recovery

— Reinforcement of the patients' responsibility for their recovery

— Practical advice on rehabilitation, exercise, and nutrition

— Detailed letter to general practitioner detailing patients' illness

— Early recognition and diagnosis of physical and psychological problems in patients and relatives

— Follow up for at least 6 months after discharge from hospital that reviews not only the patient's physical problems but also psychological issues for patients and close relatives

It is helpful to outline a plan with patients and their families for convalescence and rehabilitation. Patients should haveaccess to referral to specialists such as clinical psychologistsand dieticians. Work, particularly in cardiac rehabilitation,suggests that providing written information about critical illness,self help advice to manage the typical problems patients mightface during recovery, and an exercise programmeme may be helpful.

Rehabilitation after Critical Illness

Early intervention is needed to prevent physical and psychological problems. This should ideally start when the patient ismoved to the ward. Activity is the key to recovery, but the overwhelmingweakness that patients report as they start to recover and thelength of the convalescent process means that they require considerabledetermination to exercise. Most patients have little idea howand when to start exercising or how to pacethemselves. Simply giving intensive care patients a discharge booklet outlining possible problems they might encounter during their recoveryhas proved unsuccessful. Despite using a booklet, 25% of patientsattending an intensive care follow up clinic scored highly foranxiety and depression 2 months after intensivecare.

EMERGENCY MEDICAL SERVICES

Emergency medical services (EMS) are critical components of the overall health care delivery system. The availability of these services to the public at large is often the only difference between life and death in a medical emergency. EMS directly affect the public's health by providing immediate intervention for victims of traumatic events, heart attacks, strokes, and motor vehicle accidents.

An estimated one in four Americans is injured annually and accounts for one in three emergency department visits.

Unintentional injuries kill 1,000 Connecticut residents and cause 36,000 hospital admissions in the state each year. Motor-vehicle-related injuries account for nearly 4,000 hospitalisations in Connecticut each year and represent 5% of emergency department visits. The more extensive discussion of injuries and their impact on Connecticut's health care system. The essential purpose of an EMS system is to reduce death and disability due to injuries and other emergent medical events. For EMS to accomplish its purpose, the system must provide for the personnel, facilities, and equipment for the efficient, effective, and coordinated delivery of health care services to handle emergencies. Typically, EMS systems incorporate 15 components — manpower, training, communications, transportation, facilities, critical care units, public safety agencies, consumer participation, access to care, transfer of patients, standardized patient record keeping, public information and education, evaluation, disaster linkages, and mutual aid agreements.

Connecticut's Emergency Medical Service System

The emergency medical services system in Connecticut is organised on three levels consisting of state, regional, and local levels. The Connecticut General Statutes identifies the responsibilities of the system to assure that each resident in the State has access to emergency medical services. Regulation of the system covers all emergency medical care providers, all personnel training requirements and authorized levels of services, all vehicle specifications and equipment standards, and the setting of rates for service delivery. Regulations are promulgated by DPH which is also responsible for the planning, development and administration of the statewide EMS system. DPH establishes minimum standards, provides technical and consulting assistance, adopts and enforces regulations, coordinates education and training programmes, prepares plans and programmes, and certifies EMS personnel and equipment. The regional level of EMS infrastructure acts as liaison between state and local efforts. Five defined EMS regions, identical to the Uniform Service Regions in Connecticut, are represented by EMS councils. These councils serve as authorized extensions of the State in performing delegated state functions and in implementing state policy and programmes at the regional and local level. The councils develop regional implementation plans that complement the state plan, provide technical assistance and serve as a voice for the local communities concerning all EMS issues.

TABLE 1

Prehospital Emergency Medical Service Providers Connecticut, 1997

Type of Provider	*Number*	*Percent*
Volunteer Fire Departments	117	42.4 %
Volunteer Ambulance Company	71	25.7 %
Private	35	12.7 %
Local Fire Department	21	7.6 %
Police Department	16	5.8 %
Hospital Based	9	3.3 %
State Institution	6	2.2 %
Municipal	1	0.3 %
Total	276	100.0 %

Source: DPH, OEMS, data compiled as of 6/30/97

The local EMS infrastructure is responsible for providing services or contracting for the needed emergency medical services in the community. The EMS delivery system includes prehospital care providers, hospital emergency departments, and specialized hospital facilities. In Connecticut, 276 commercial, municipal, or volunteer providers served the public's need for prehospital emergency medical services in 1997. Over 40% of these providers are volunteer fire departments and one-quarter are volunteer ambulance companies. The hospital emergency departments in Connecticut are dedicated to offering emergency medical evaluation and initial treatment to patients. When an injury requires advanced patient care as a result of a serious injury or illness, the victim may best be served in a facility that offers specialized emergency care 24 hours a day such as a trauma center, burn center, neonatal or pediatric center. There are nine Connecticut hospitals that are designated as trauma facilities and serve as participants in the EMS trauma delivery system (Table 2).

TABLE 2

Designated Trauma Facilities
Connecticut, 1997

Trauma Level and Hospital	
Level I[a]	
	Bridgeport Hospital
	Hartford Hospital
	St. Francis Hospital and Medical Center
	Yale New Haven Hospital
Level II[b]	
	Hospital of Saint Raphael
	St. Mary's Hospital
	St. Vincent's Hospital
	Stamford Hospital
	Waterbury Hospital

Source: DPH, OEMS, data compiled as of 4/23/97.

(a) Level I indicates comprehensive emergency services offering complete and advanced patient care for all emergencies including those requiring complex and specialized emergency care 24 hours a day.

(b) Level II offers advanced patient care in all medical and surgical specialties to render resuscitation and life-support 24 hours a day.

The EMS delivery system involves both the public and private sector working together to provide the necessary services to meet the emergency medical needs of our residents. The variety of stakeholders range from a small local fire department to the large city hospital, but each is involved in this critical component of the overall health care delivery system in Connecticut.

EMS Relationship with *Healthy Connecticut 2000*

Emergency medical services contribute towards the state's achievement of year 2000 goals. Objective 1.1 of *Healthy Connecticut 2000* is to reduce coronary heart disease deaths to no more than 84/100,000 people. The presence and expertise of EMS personnel who are trained in cardiopulmonary resuscitation and advanced cardiac care can provide direct intervention for reducing coronary heart disease deaths. *Healthy Connecticut 2000* identifies objectives for reducing violence that results in death and disability, and *Healthy Connecticut 2000* relates to unintentional injury objectives such as reducing deaths from motor vehicle crashes, falls, drownings, and residential fires. Emergency medical services are often the first medical care provided to victims of violence and injuries. Thus, the service is critical for reducing death and disability outcomes as identified in *Healthy Connecticut 2000*.

Connecticut EMS Plan

In January of 1997, the DPH published the latest statewide EMS plan. The plan identifies the need for a uniform funding mechanism, the lack of a statewide prehospital data collection system, and the need to designate primary service area responders for all levels of service (i.e. first responder, basic ambulance, and paramedic). Public health professionals need adequate information to develop, implement, and evaluate prevention programmes, and decision makers need timely information to develop policies to prevent injuries and unintentional deaths. Baseline and follow-up studies of trauma incidence and outcomes are instrumental in planning, implementing, and evaluating a trauma care system. Among the most useful data sources are trauma registries, hospital discharge data, vital statistics, EMS run reports, and surveys that assess hospital trauma care capabilities.

DPH, in collaboration with the Connecticut Hospital Association, developed a trauma registry that identifies traumatic injuries; however, there is no mechanism to evaluate the overall EMS system, its effectiveness of services, and the appropriateness of care provided to victims of medical and trauma related emergencies. DPH has revised an EMS "run form" to collect information about emergency medical services and is available to all providers free of charge. The form has not been widely used and there is no requirement for providers to submit the information to the State. Each EMS service, in cooperation with its sponsoring hospital, determines which "run form" it will use and what additional data beyond the minimum is to be included. Therefore, there are multiple forms that are not compatible between regions, municipalities, or hospital service areas. There is an effort underway to develop a prehospital data base that can link to the trauma registry and the hospital discharge data base to assess and evaluate the continuity of care for medical emergency victims. DPH has drafted a scope of work and is in the process of developing a data management system to collect and analyse data when contributed. This is in response to the goals and objectives outlined in the EMS plan. The objectives in the state EMS Plan are considered ambitious but necessary to be prepared for an increasing demand for emergency medical resources. The conditions that are present now will be present in the future and increase with a rapidly aging population. The increasing incidence of violent crime in the urban areas and the spread of diverse infectious diseases inspires the EMS system to respond appropriately. It is one of the few health care services that is relied upon so heavily by the entire population. Current and proposed efforts to improve the system may require budget assessments and reallocations and redefined priorities at the local, regional, state, and federal levels.

HEALTH AND SAFETY PARAMEDIC AND OTHER EMERGENCY MEDICAL SERVICE SYSTEMS, EMERGENCY MEDICAL SERVICES SYSTEMS

Purposes

The purposes of the emergency medical services systems legislation are to establish and/or identify specific roles and responsibilities in regard to emergency medical services in Delaware in order to reduce morbidity and mortality rates for the citizens of Delaware and to ensure quality of emergency care services, within available resources, through the effective coordination of the emergency medical services system.

Definitions

As used in this subchapter:

1. "Advanced life support" (ALS) shall mean the advanced level of prehospital and interhospital emergency care that includes basic life support functions including cardiopulmonary resuscitation, plus cardiac monitoring, cardiac defibrillation, telemetered electrocardiography, administration of antiarrhythmic agents, intravenous therapy, administration of specific medications, drugs and solutions, use of adjunctive medical devices, trauma care and other authorized techniques and procedures.
2. "Ambulance" shall mean any publicly or privately

owned vehicle, as certified by the State Fire Prevention Commission, that is specifically designed, constructed or modified and equipped, and is intended to be used for and is maintained or operated for the transportation upon the streets and highways of this State for persons who are sick, injured, wounded or otherwise incapacitated or helpless.

3. "Ambulance attendant" shall mean a person trained in emergency medical care procedures and currently certified by the Delaware State Fire Prevention Commission or its duly authorized agent in accordance with standards prescribed by the Commission. Such course shall be classified as basic life support and shall be the minimum acceptable level of training for certified emergency medical personnel.
4. "Basic life support" (BLS) shall mean the level of capability which provides prehospital, noninvasive emergency patient care designed to optimize the patient's chances of surviving an emergency situation.
5. "Consumer" shall mean a recipient or potential recipient of the services provided by an emergency medical services system, who receives no direct or indirect personal, financial or professional benefit as a result of association with health care or emergency services other than that generally shared by the public at large, and who is not otherwise considered a "provider" within the intent of this subchapter.
6. "Director" shall mean the programme chief of the Office of Emergency Medical Services responsible for the duties of the Office.
7. "Disaster" shall mean a sudden unexpected event which disrupts normal community functions and/or

quickly exhausts local facilities so as to require outside help.

8. "Early defibrillation provider" shall mean a member or employee of an early defibrillation service certified to operate Semi-Automatic External Defibrillator (SAED) equipment under the requirements set forth in regulations promulgated by the Department of Health and Social Services.
9. "Early defibrillation service" shall mean any agency, organisation or company, certified as such by the State Office of Emergency Medical Services, that employs or retains providers certified in the use of semi-automatic defibrillation equipment.
10. "Emergency medical services systems" (EMSS) shall mean a statewide system which provides for the utilisation of available personnel, equipment, transportation and communication to ensure effective and coordinated delivery of medical care in emergency situations resulting from accidents, illness or natural disasters.
11. "Emergency medical technician" (EMT) shall mean a person trained, and currently certified by the State Fire Prevention Commission, in emergency medical care procedures through a course which meets the objectives of the national standard curriculum.
12. "Emergency medical technician — cardiac" (EMT-C), also known as cardiac rescue technician (CRT), shall mean a person who has successfully completed a course approved by the Board of Medical Practice or its duly authorized representative, which meets the objectives of the national standard curriculum.
13. "Emergency medical technician — paramedic" (EMT-P) shall mean a person who has successfully

completed a course approved by the Board of Medical Practice or its duly authorized representative, and who acts under the direct or radio control of a physician or physician surrogate.

14. "Health planning agencies" shall mean the federally designated health system agency and/or statewide health planning and development agency for Delaware.
15. "Inclusive Statewide Trauma Care System" means a Trauma System in which all current and future providers of hospital and/or prehospital health care services may participate, at a level commensurate with the scope of their resources, as outlined in subsection (21) of this section.
16. "Medical control" shall mean directions and advice normally provided from a centrally designated medical facility operating under medical supervision, supplying professional support through radio or telephonic communication for on-site and in-transit basic and advanced life support services given by field and satellite facility personnel.
17. "Mutual aid agreements" shall mean the establishment of appropriate arrangements with EMS systems of other states for the provision of emergency medical services on a reciprocal basis.
18. "Provider" shall mean a person who, as an individual or member of a corporation or organisation, whether profit-making or nonprofit, on a regular basis gives or offers for sale any supplies, equipment, professional or nonprofessional services, or is capable of giving or offering for sale supplies, equipment or services vital or incidental to the functions of an emergency medical services system.
19. "Public safety personnel" shall mean law-enforcement

officers, lifeguards, park rangers, firefighters, ambulance and rescue personnel, communications and dispatch specialists and other public employees and emergency service providers charged with maintaining the public safety.

20. "Semi-automatic external defibrillator" shall mean a device capable of analysing a cardiac rhythm, determining the need for defibrillation, automatically charging and advising a provider to deliver a defibrillation electrical impulse.
21. "Specialty care unit" shall mean sophisticated treatment facilities that provide advanced specialized definitive care for critically ill patients. The units shall be available for the diagnosis and care of specific patient problems including major trauma, burns, spinal cord injury, poisoning, acute cardiac, high-risk infant and behavioural emergencies.
22. "Trauma Facility" means an acute care hospital which has received and maintains current State designation as a Trauma Center. Categories of trauma facilities in Delaware are as follows:
    (a) Regional Level 1 Trauma Center: A regional resource Trauma Center that has the capability of providing leadership and comprehensive, definitive care for every aspect of injury from prevention through rehabilitation.
    (b) Regional Level 2 Trauma Center: A regional Trauma Center with the capability to provide initial care for all trauma patients. Most patients would continue to be cared for in this Center; there may be some complex cases which would require transfer for the depth of services of a Regional Level 1 or Specialty Center.

(c) Community Trauma Center: An acute care hospital that provides assessment, resuscitation, stabilisation and triage of all trauma patients, arranging for timely transfer of those patients requiring the additional resources of a Regional Trauma or Specialty Center and delivering definitive care to those whose needs match the resources of the Community Trauma Center.

(d) Participating Hospital: An acute care facility which transfers trauma patients with moderate or severe injuries to Trauma Centers after initial resuscitation. When necessary, this facility may provide care to trauma patients with minor injuries. Participating hospitals contribute data to the Delaware Trauma System Registry and Quality Improvement Programme.

23. "Trauma Patient" means any person with actual or potential bodily damage subsequent to an event which exposed the body to an external force or energy.

24. "Treatment protocols" shall mean written uniform treatment and care plans for emergency and critical patients. The treatment plans for advanced life support must be approved and signed by appropriate physicians and/or medical groups.

Delaware Emergency Medical Services Oversight Council

(a) There is established the Delaware Emergency Medical Services Oversight Council (DEMSOC). The Council shall consist of the following members:

1. A representative of the Office of the Governor appointed by the Governor:
2. The Secretary of the Department of Safety and Homeland Security;

3. The Secretary of the Department of Health and Social Services, or at the discretion of the Secretary, the Director of Public Health;
4. The Chair of the Delaware State Fire Prevention Commission or another Commissioner selected by the Chair;
5. The President of the Delaware Volunteer Fireman's Association;
6. he Colonel of the New Castle County Police Department or, at the Colonel's discretion, the Director of New Castle County Emergency Medical Services;
7. The Kent County Administrator or, at the Administrator's discretion, the Kent County EMS Chief;
8. The Sussex County Administrator, or at the Administrator's discretion, the Sussex County EMS Director;
9. The President of the Delaware Chapter of the American College of Emergency Physicians;
10. The State EMS Medical Director;
11. The Chair of the Trauma Systems Committee;
12. A practicing paramedic, certified and employed in the State, appointed by the Governor;
13. The Chair of the DVFA Ambulance Advisory Committee;
14. Three additional at-large members, 1 from each county, appointed by the Governor; and
15. The President of the Delaware Healthcare Association or, at the President's discretion, a representative of the Delaware Healthcare Association.
16. The Executive Director of the Medical Society of Delaware or, at the Executive Director's discretion,

a representative of the Medical Society of Delaware; and

17. The Chair of the Delaware Police Chiefs' Council or, at the Chair's discretion, a representative of the Delaware Police Chief's Council.
18. The Paramedic Commander of the Delaware State Police Aviation Unit.

(b) The members of the Council may designate a voting alternate representative.

(c) The Council shall meet at a minimum of 1 time per year.

(d) The Chairperson of the Council shall be designated from among the members by the Governor and shall serve at the pleasure of the Governor. The Chairperson shall select a Vice Chairperson from the membership of the Council to serve in the Chairperson's absence.

(e) The Council shall monitor Delaware's emergency medical services system to ensure that all elements of the system are functioning in a coordinated, effective, and efficient manner in order to reduce morbidity and mortality rates for the citizens of Delaware and to ensure quality of emergency care services.

(f) The Council shall have the following duties and responsibilities:

(1) To examine policies and procedures and evaluate the effectiveness of the EMS system, specifically the respective roles, responsibilities, effectiveness and efficiency of the Office of Emergency Medical Services (OEMS), the State Fire Prevention Commission, the Department of Safety and

Homeland Security, the EMS provider agencies and the medical community;

(2) To study, research, plan, evaluate as well as offer guidance to, cooperate with and assist public agencies and private institutions and organisations on methods for the coordination and effective utilisation of their emergency medical service programmes;

(3) To formulate goals and recommendations, based on objective criteria and data, to be used in evaluating EMS provider agency performance;

(4) To review and make recommendations concerning quality improvement efforts pursuant to this chapter;

(5) To make recommendations to the Office of EMS, the Department of Safety and Homeland Security, the EMS provider agencies and the medical community for improving EMS in Delaware;

(6) To make legislative recommendations to the Governor and General Assembly;

(7) To provide an annual report on or before April 15 of each year to the Governor, General Assembly, interested parties and the public which will outline the performance of all EMS system agencies, comparing that performance to established goals and performance measures. The report shall also estimate the costs of Delaware's EMS medical system. Automatic external defibrillator and cardio-pulmonary resuscitation programme performance shall be included in this report.

The first report will cover service provided in calendar year 2000 and will be delivered by April 15, 2001;

(8) To make recommendations concerning EMS to the State Fire Prevention Commission. The Commission will consider and act upon those recommendations; and

(9) To conduct a full review of EMS in the State at a minimum of every 5 years.

(g) The Council may request and shall receive from any department, division, commission or agency of the State such reasonable assistance and data as will enable it to properly carry out its functions hereunder.

(h) OEMS shall staff the Council.

Office of Emergency Medical Services — Created; Purpose

(a) The Office of Emergency Medical Services is hereby created. The Office shall be responsible for ensuring the effective coordination and evaluation of the emergency medical services system in Delaware which includes providing assistance and advice for activities related toward the planning, development, improvement and expansion of emergency medical services.

(b) The Office of Emergency Medical Services shall be a state agency within the Division of Public Health, Department of Health and Social Services. The Office of Emergency Medical Services shall report directly to and be responsible to the Director of the Division of Public Health, which is consistent with the health plan for Delaware.

(c) As used in this subchapter, the term "Office" shall refer to the State Office of Emergency Medical Services. In the performance of the functions mandated by this legislation which relate to the planning and evaluation of the emergency medical services system in Delaware, the Office of Emergency Medical Services shall coordinate with the Bureau of Health Planning and Resources Development for technical assistance in emergency medical services planning activities. Specifically, the Bureau of Health Planning and Resources Development shall have the primary responsibility for all data analysis related to the emergency medical services system. This coordination should minimize duplication of effort between the 2 agencies and allow for the effective use of available staff resources within the Department of Health and Social Services.

(d) Except for those activities and responsibilities for basic life support, which are under the jurisdiction of the State Fire Prevention Commission, the Office of Emergency Medical Services shall have jurisdiction over the development, implementation and maintenance of a Statewide Trauma System.

(e) A memorandum of agreement shall be established between the Office of Emergency Medical Services of the Division of Public Health and the State Fire Prevention Commission to foster inclusion and coordination of Basic Life Support Services within the Statewide Trauma System.

(f) The Director of Public Health shall establish a standing Trauma System Committee and ad hoc committees as deemed appropriate to assist in oversight of the Inclusive Statewide Trauma Care System. The standing Trauma System Committee shall convene at least quarterly. Membership on the standing Trauma System Committee will include, but not be limited to, a representative of each of the following constituencies to be selected from the 3 counties within the State:

1. Trauma rehabilitation professionals

2. Practicing trauma surgeons
3. Practicing emergency department physicians
4. The Association of Delaware Hospitals
5. Advanced Life Support prehospital providers
6. Basic Life Support prehospital providers
7. The State Fire School
8. Practicing trauma subspecialty physicians
9. Practicing pediatric surgeons or pediatricians
10. Practicing registered nurses involved in trauma patient care
11. Emergency medical dispatchers
12. Hospital administration
13. The Delaware state police aviation section
14. A representative from the State Fire Prevention Commission.

(g) The Trauma System Committee shall be an advisory group to the Director of Public Health on the following issues:

1. Rules governing the operation of Delaware's Inclusive Statewide Trauma Care System, which will be based upon national references such as the American College of Surgeons' Resources for Optimal Care of the Trauma Patient: 1993.
2. Recommendations for corrective action based on the reviews of the following:
   (a) Statewide trauma care system operations, including the monitoring for adherence to adopted policies, procedures, protocols and standards, the availability of appropriate resources and the periodic review of trauma hospital participation (designation) criteria.
   (b) The delivery of emergency medical and hospital

services by trauma care service providers to trauma patients.

3. Recommendation for modifications of the policies, procedures and protocols of trauma care as a result of system-wide review.

Office of Emergency Medical Services — Functions

(a) Personnel. — It shall be the responsibility of the Office to collect and analyse annually data pertaining to certified emergency medical services personnel in Delaware by levels of training in order to identify possible or potential shortages. Once EMS personnel shortages are identified, the Office shall notify the affected agencies and provide recommended courses of action to alleviate the problem or potential problem. In order to accomplish this task, the following agencies shall be required to provide a listing of the appropriate emergency medical services personnel by organisation, level of training and county:

1. Delaware State Fire Prevention Commission or its duly authorized representative;
2. Wilmington Medical Center School for Emergency Medical Technicians;
3. Delaware Committee on Trauma of the American College of Surgeons — advanced trauma life support;
4. American Heart Association of Delaware — cardiopulmonary resuscitation (CPR) training programmes and advanced cardiac life support;
5. American Red Cross, Delaware Chapter — CPR training and first-aid training;
6. Delaware Chapter of the American College of Emergency Physicians;
7. Delaware Chapter of the Emergency Department Nurses Association; and

8. Any other organisation not listed above that provides certified emergency medical training, including CPR.

(b) Training. — All organisations providing emergency medical training programmes, as listed under the personnel section, shall provide to the Office copies of course curricula and schedules of the availability of training courses. The Office shall monitor EMS training levels to provide information on the availability of training programmes for all levels of EMS personnel. In addition, the EMS Office shall keep abreast of all federal training standards to ensure that EMS training agencies in Delaware are aware of regional and national standards. In accordance with § 6711(a)(3) [repealed] of this title, the State Fire Prevention Commission shall adopt regulations setting forth the qualifications required for the certification of ambulance attendants. Since advanced life support ambulance personnel are "physicians' assistants" They must have been trained in programmes approved by the Delaware State Board of Medical Practice.

(c) Communications. — The Office shall:

1. Through the appropriate county dispatch center directors, monitor and evaluate the effectiveness of the statewide EMS communications system;
2. Identify resources to improve or augment both the communications system in Delaware and the training of medical dispatchers as needed;
3. Monitor and evaluate the effectiveness of emergency access numbers in terms of the impact on the EMS system.

(d) Transportation. — In conjunction with appropriate EMS providers in Delaware, the Office shall monitor and evaluate emergency medical transportation services in Delaware to ensure that patients in the EMS system have access to effective and efficient transportation to appropriate treatment facilities. Pursuant to § 6709 of this title, all ambulances in Delaware shall be inspected and certified by the Delaware State Fire Prevention Commission or a duly authorized representative thereof. The Delaware State Fire Prevention Commission or its duly authorized representative shall be required to provide to the Office on an annual basis a listing and location of certified ambulances.

(e) Facilities. — The Office shall monitor the availability of the various levels of care of EMS facilities and services and shall have the authority to categorize all Delaware emergency receiving facilities and services in accordance with criteria established by the Joint Commission on Accreditation of Hospitals (JCAH) for hospital settings and other appropriate national professional organisations for nonhospital settings. This authority shall also include the responsibility of categorizing and designating by level of care, when appropriate, specialty care facilities in accordance with the established criteria of the American Medical Association or other appropriate national professional organisations. In addition, the Office shall periodically re-evaluate the categorisation or designation of emergency care facilities and specialty care services.

(f) Specialty care units. — The Office shall identify the categorisation of the 7 specialty care areas for EMS which are available to all patients (the specialty care areas are: Trauma, burns, spinal cord, poisoning, acute cardiac, high-risk infant and behavioural emergencies). In addition, the Office shall coordinate the activities of the EMS system to ensure that all patients have access, within a reasonable time period depending on the nature of the illness, to specialty care services. In accordance with this activity, the Office shall have the authority to designate or categorize specialty care units by level of care as specified in the section related to facilities.

(g) Public safety agencies. — Based on the data obtained in the section related to personnel, the Office shall monitor and evaluate the activities of public safety agencies to determine the number of trained first responders and to promote their participation, to the maximum level possible consistent with their capabilities, in emergency medical situations.

(h) Consumer participation. — All agencies and organisations involved in the EMS system in Delaware should seek reasonable consumer participation in planning, development and organisational activities.

(i) Access to care. — The Office shall monitor and evaluate activities of all EMS organisations to ensure that no person is denied emergency treatment or transportation services.

(j) Patient transfer. — The EMS system shall provide for transfer of patients to facilities and programmes which offer such follow-up care and rehabilitation as is necessary to effect the maximum recovery of the patient. The transfer of emergency patients from the emergency site to the emergency department, specialty care unit and to follow-up care and rehabilitation centers are all within the scope of a total EMS system.

(k) Coordinated patient recordkeeping. — The Office shall collect and analyse available data from all providers of the EMS system. This data will be used by the Office, in conjunction with the appropriate EMS providers, to evaluate the overall effectiveness of the system. It is necessary that the data be collected from each level of care, which includes the initial entry point through final discharge from the health care delivery system. EMS agency certification will be contingent upon agency participation in the Statewide EMS data collection system maintained by the Office.

(l) Public information, prevention and education. —

The Office shall provide programmes of public information and education designed to inform residents of Delaware and visitors to the State of the availability of, proper use of and access to emergency medical services. The Office shall also support prevention activities designed to address key categories of illness and injury as identified through data collection. The Office will serve as a clearinghouse for illness and injury prevention activity, and will work to coordinate EMS prevention efforts statewide. These programmes shall include elements related to citizen involvement in the administration of prehospital care, such as cardiopulmonary resuscitation and first aid, and information concerning the availability of training programmes in Delaware. In addition, the Office shall monitor public information and education programmes offered by other EMS providers in Delaware. All EMS provider agencies shall provide a report on their prevention and education activities conducted during the previous year to the Office by January 15 of each year. The Office shall publish an annual report outlining the status of prevention and public education activities throughout the State by May 15 of each year.

(m) Review and evaluation. — In conjunction with the health planning agencies and the EMS providers in Delaware, the Office shall conduct and/or coordinate an on-going comprehensive evaluation of the effectiveness of the EMS system, in terms of the impact on the health status of the EMS patients in Delaware.

(n) Disaster planning. — The Office shall: (1) Upon request, participate in disaster planning with all organisations that provide emergency medical services to assist with coordination of disaster activities which impact the EMS system, and (2) review all municipal, county and state disaster plans which utilize the emergency medical services system. All organisations involved in planning disaster exercises which impact the EMS system should advise the Office of scheduled disaster exercises. In addition, the Office shall, upon request, participate in disaster exercises for the purpose of evaluation and improvement of the emergency medical services system and make recommendations as needed to the appropriate provider for the refinement of their disaster plans. All disaster planning activities of the Office shall be coordinated with the Delaware Emergency Management Agency as authorized, and the Department of Health and Social Services Disaster Coordinator.

(o) Mutual aid agreements. — The Director of the Office in conjunction with the Division Director shall be authorized to develop and implement mutual aid agreements as may be necessary to ensure continuity of care. These agreements shall be coordinated through and approved by the appropriate EMS providers. These agreements may relate to reciprocity of services, and treatment, transfer and triage protocols to coordinate the provision of services, both within Delaware and across state lines as necessary.

(p) Semi-automatic external defibrillators. —

1. The Department of Health and Social Services shall promulgate regulations specific to the use of semi-automatic external defibrillators and shall seek input and review from the Board of Medical Practice, the Delaware EMS Oversight Council and the Delaware State Fire Prevention Commission.
2. The Office shall coordinate a statewide effort to promote and implement widespread use of semi-automatic external defibrillators and cardio-pulmonary resuscitation to increase the number of publicly available SAEDs to 100 by January 1, 2002, and 200 by January 1, 2004. In addition, the Office shall coordinate a statewide effort to provide, train

and maintain a minimum of 5 qualified individuals for each publicly available SAED.

3. All law enforcement vehicles on patrol shall be equipped with a semi-automatic external defibrillator by January 1, 2001, subject to appropriations.

Office of Emergency Medical Services — Additional functions

(a) In order to monitor and evaluate the effectiveness of the EMS system, the Office must be notified of any proposed new service or major service modification within the emergency medical services system in Delaware.

(b) Copies of applications for federal, state and county emergency medical service grant funds shall be sent to the Office.

(c) All proposed legislation pertaining to the EMS system in Delaware shall be reviewed by DEMSOC with recommendations from the Office.

(d) The Office shall, with the consent of the Director of the Division of Public Health, be authorized to make news releases pertaining to the emergency medical services system as required in order to inform the public on issues pertinent to the health and well being of the citizens of Delaware.

(e) The Office shall be required to provide routine progress reports identifying the accomplishments and the problem areas within the system to DEMSOC at its regularly scheduled meetings. In addition, an annual summary report shall be sent to the Chairperson of DEMSOC through the Division Director by August 15 of each year.

(f) The Office is authorized and empowered to apply for, accept and disburse grants, gifts and contributions from the government, individuals, foundations, corporations and other organisations, agencies or institutions on behalf of the EMS system in Delaware.

(g) The Director of Public Health shall, except for those activities and responsibilities for basic life support, which is under the jurisdiction of the State Fire Prevention Commission:

1. Use the Trauma System Committee recommendations as the basis for establishing a plan for the implementation and maintenance of Delaware's Inclusive Statewide Trauma Care System. The State Trauma System Plan shall address each component of trauma care as outlined in national references such as Model Trauma Care System Plan, HRSA-BHRD, September 1990 and subsequent revisions. These include, but are not limited to:
   (a) Prehospital care — Standardized and statewide policies, procedure and protocols to be used by all emergency medical service providers and licensed personnel for the identification, treatment and transport of trauma patients.
   (b) Prevention — Efforts to decrease the numbers and severity of injuries, resulting in decreased demand for care.
   (c) Hospital care — Standards and criteria for hospital personnel, equipment and designation that identify the necessary resources that hospitals must have in order to be recognized within Delaware's Inclusive Statewide Trauma Care System as a specified category trauma facility. These standards and criteria shall be consistent with those identified in national trauma system references, such as the American College of Surgeons' Resources for Optimal Care of the Injured Patient: 1993 and subsequent revisions. All expenses associated with utilizing a nationally recognized accreditation team to

verify a hospital's compliance with hospital designation criteria will be the responsibility of the hospital being surveyed.

(d) Rehabilitative care — Standards for the follow-up care for persons with disabilities resulting from injuries.

(e) Trauma continuing education — The on-going trauma related education for trauma care system personnel/providers to maintain knowledge and skills.

(f) Trauma care system evaluation — Monitor policies and procedures regarding the effectiveness/impact of trauma care systems.

2. The Director of Public Health shall have the authority to promulgate rules for the management of all components of Delaware's Inclusive Statewide Trauma Care System, and shall seek input and review from the Trauma System Committee.
3. Maintain a programme of trauma care system evaluation, including a trauma data collection and registry system and a mechanism for evaluating and monitoring system performance throughout the continuum of trauma care.

(h) The Director of Public Health shall have the authority to promulgate rules for EMS provider recognition and compliance with an advanced health care directive that has become effective pursuant to § 2503(c) of this title, and shall seek input and review from the Board of Medical Practice, the Delaware EMS Advisory Council and the Delaware State Fire Prevention Commission. For purposes of this subsection, "EMS provider" shall mean providers certified by the Delaware State Fire Commission or the Office of Emergency Medical Services within the Division of Public Health, Department of Health and Social Services. EMS providers acting in accordance with the regulations promulgated hereunder shall be immune from criminal or civil liability pursuant to § 2510 of this title.

1. The regulation shall define prehospital advanced care directive procedures to be used for terminally ill patients only.
2. All sections of the regulation will insure that processes are in compliance of this title, the "Delaware Death with Dignity Act." The regulations shall include, but not be limited to, the following:
   (a) The allowable content of prehospital advanced care directives, to include:
      (1) Option A (Advanced Life Support) — Maximal (Restorative) Care Before Arrest, then prehospital advanced care directive; or
      (2) Option B (Basic Life Support) — Limited (Palliative) Care Only Before Arrest, then prehospital advanced care directive;
   (b) Methods of identification describing the methods that can be used by persons electing to enact a prehospital advanced care directive. The properly enacted Delaware Prehospital Advanced Care Directive Form must be present; however, voluntary use of a Medic Alert prehospital advanced care directive bracelet or necklace may be worn and/or a designation on a person's driver's license or state-issued identification card pursuant to § 2718(c) of Title 21 to indicate the presence of the form;
   (c) Methods of revocation of prehospital advanced care directive describing how a prehospital

advanced care directive can be revoked of this title; and

(d) Reciprocity to allow Delaware EMS providers to recognize prehospital advanced care directives from neighboring states for persons in Delaware.

Confidentiality of Quality Review Programme and Participants.

(a) Confidentiality of quality review programme and participants. — As used in this section, "records" means the recordings of interviews and all oral or written reports, statements, minutes, memoranda, charts, statistics, data and other documentation generated by the Trauma System Committee or its subcommittees for the stated purposes of trauma system medical review or quality care review and audit.

All quality management proceedings shall be confidential. Records of the Trauma System Committee, its quality care review committee and members, attendees and visitors at meetings held for stated purposes of trauma system medical review or quality care review and audit shall be confidential and privileged and shall be protected from direct or indirect means of discovery, subpoena or admission into evidence in any judicial or administrative proceeding. Raw data shall not be available for public inspection nor is it a public record within the meaning of the Delaware Freedom of Information Act.

(b) Confidentiality of Delaware Emergency Medical Services Oversight Council (DEMSOC) quality review programme and participants. — As used in this section, "records" means the recordings of interviews and all oral or written reports, statements, minutes, memoranda, charts, statistics, data and other documentation generated by the Delaware Emergency Medical Services Oversight Council (DEMSOC) or its subcommittees for the stated purposes of the Emergency Medical Services System medical review or quality care review and audit. All quality management proceedings shall be confidential. Records of DEMSOC, its quality care review subcommittees and members, attendees and visitors at meetings held for stated purposes of the Emergency Medical Services Systems medical review or quality care review and audit shall not be available for public inspection nor are they a public record within the meaning of the Delaware Freedom of Information Act, and shall be protected from direct or indirect means of discovery, subpoena or admission into evidence in any judicial or administrative proceeding. Raw data and original records relating to medical care shall not be available for public inspection nor are they a public record within the meaning of the Delaware Freedom of Information Act, except to the extent that such raw data and original records relating to medical care would have been subject to disclosure or discovery pursuant to other statute or court rule.

(c) Immunity. — No person shall be subject to, and shall be immune from, any claim, suit, liability, damages or any other recourse, civil or criminal, arising from any act or proceeding, decision or determination undertaken or performed, or recommendation made while discharging any duty or authority under this chapter, so long as such person acted in good faith without malice, and within the scope of his or her duty or authority under this chapter or any other provisions of the Delaware law, federal law or regulations or duly adopted rules and regulations providing for the administration of this chapter, good faith being presumed until proven otherwise, with malice required to be shown by the complainant.

OPTIONAL HOSPITAL SERVICES

Condition of Participation: Surgical Services

If the hospital provides surgical services, the services must be well organised and provided in accordance with acceptable standards of practice. If outpatient surgical services are offered the services must be consistent in quality with inpatient care in accordance with the complexity of services offered.

(a) *Standard: Organisation and staffing.* The organisation of the surgical services must be appropriate to the scope of the services offered.

1. The operating rooms must be supervised by an experienced registered nurse or a doctor of medicine or osteopathy.
2. Licensed practical nurses (LPNs) and surgical technologists (operating room technicians) may serve as "scrub nurses" under the supervision of a registered nurse.
3. Qualified registered nurses may perform circulating duties in the operating room. In accordance with applicable State laws and approved medical staff policies and procedures, LPNs and surgical technologists may assist in circulatory duties under the surpervision of a qualified registered nurse who is immediately available to respond to emergencies.
4. Surgical privileges must be delineated for all practitioners performing surgery in accordance with the competencies of each practitioner. The surgical service must maintain a roster of practitioners specifying the surgical privileges of each practitioner.

(b) *Standard: Delivery of service.* Surgical services must be consistent with needs and resources. Policies governing surgical care must be designed to assure the achievement and maintenance of high standards of medical practice and patient care.

1. There must be a complete history and physical work-up in the chart of every patient prior to surgery, except in emergencies. If this has been dictated, but not yet recorded in the patient's chart, there must be a statement to that effect and an admission note in the chart by the practitioner who admitted the patient.
2. A properly executed informed consent form for the operation must be in the patient's chart before surgery, except in emergencies.
3. The following equipment must be available to the operating room suites: call-in-system, cardiac monitor, resuscitator, defibrillator, aspirator, and tracheotomy set.
4. There must be adequate provisions for immediate post-operative care.
5. The operating room register must be complete and up-to-date.
6. An operative report describing techniques, findings, and tissues removed or altered must be written or dictated immediately following surgery and signed by the surgeon.

Condition of Participation: Anesthesia Services

If the hospital furnishes anesthesia services, they must be provided in a well-organised manner under the direction of a qualified doctor of medicine or osteopathy. The service is responsible for all anesthesia administered in the hospital.

(a) *Standard: Organisation and staffing.* The organisation of anesthesia services must be appropriate to the scope of the services offered. Anesthesia must be administered only by—

1. A qualified anesthesiologist;
2. A doctor of medicine or osteopathy (other than an anesthesiologist);
3. A dentist, oral surgeon, or podiatrist who is qualified to administer anesthesia under State law;
4. A certified registered nurse anesthetist (CRNA), as defined, who, unless exempted in accordance with paragraph of this section, is under the supervision of the operating practitioner or of an anesthesiologist who is immediately available if needed; or
5. An anesthesiologist's assistant, who is under the supervision of an anesthesiologist who is immediately available if needed.

(b) *Standard: Delivery of services.* Anesthesia services must be consistent with needs and resources. Policies on anesthesia procedures must include the delineation of preanesthesia and post anesthesia responsibilities. The policies must ensure that the following are provided for each patient:

1. A preanesthesia evaluation by an individual qualified to administer anesthesia under paragraph (a) of this section performed within 48 hours prior to surgery.
2. An intraoperative anesthesia record.
3. With respect to inpatients, a postanesthesia followup report by the individual who administers the anesthesia that is written within 48 hours after surgery.

4. With respect to outpatients, a postanesthesia evaluation for proper anesthesia recovery performed in accordance with policies and procedures approved by the medical staff.

(c) *Standard: State exemption.*

(1) A hospital may be exempted from the requirement for physician supervision of CRNAs as described in paragraph (a) (4) of this section, if the State in which the hospital is located submits a letter to CMS signed by the Governor, following consultation with the State's Boards of Medicine and Nursing, requesting exemption from physician supervision of CRNAs. The letter from the Governor must attest that he or she has consulted with State Boards of Medicine and Nursing about issues related to access to and the quality of anesthesia services in the State and has concluded that it is in the best interests of the State's citizens to optout of the current physician supervision requirement, and that the optout is consistent with State law.

2. The request for exemption and recognition of State laws, and the withdrawal of the request may be submitted at any time, and are effective upon submission.

[51 FR 22042, June 17, 1986 as amended at 57 FR 33900, July 31, 1992; 66 FR 56769, Nov. 13, 2001]

Condition of Participation: Nuclear Medicine Services

If the hospital provides nuclear medicine services, those services must meet the needs of the patients in accordance with acceptable standards of practice.

(a) *Standard: Organisation and staffing.* The

organisation of the nuclear medicine service must be appropriate to the scope and complexity of the services offered.

1. There must be a director who is a doctor of medicine or osteopathy qualified in nuclear medicine.
2. The qualifications, training, functions, and responsibilities of nuclear medicine personnel must be specified by the service director and approved by the medical staff.

(b) *Standard: Delivery of service.* Radioactive materials must be prepared, labeled, used, transported, stored, and disposed of in accordance with acceptable standards of practice.

1. In-house preparation of radiopharmaceuticals is by, or under, the direct supervision of an appropriately trained registered pharmacist or a doctor of medicine or osteopathy.
2. There is proper storage and disposal of radioactive material.
3. If laboratory tests are performed in the nuclear medicine service, the service must meet the applicable requirement for laboratory services specified in §482.27.

(c) *Standard: Facilities.* Equipment and supplies must be appropriate for the types of nuclear medicine services offered and must be maintained for safe and efficient performance.

FIELD HOSPITAL

A field hospital is a large mobile medical unit that temporarily takes care of casualties on-site before they can be safely transported to more permanent hospital facilities. The concept was inherited from the battlefield (such as the MASH: mobile army surgical hospital), and is now applied in case of disasters or massive accidents, as well as the traditional military usage.

A field hospital is a medical staff with a mobile medical kit and, often, a wide tent-like shelter (at times an inflatable structure in modern usage) so it can be readily set up near the source of the casualties. In an urban environment, the field hospital is often established in an easily accessible and highly visible building (e.g. restaurant, school, etc.). In case of an airborne structure, the mobile medical kit is often placed in normalized container; the container itself is then used as shelter.

MEDICAL LABORATORY

A medical laboratory or clinical laboratory is a laboratory where tests are done on biological specimens in order to get information about the health of a patient.

Departments

The laboratory is often divided into a number of disciplines:

- Microbiology receive swabs, feces, urine, blood, sputum, medical equipment, as well as possible infected tissue. They culture this to check for any pathogenic microbes.
- Hematology receive whole blood and citrated plasma. They do full blood counts, blood films and coagulation investigations.
- Biochemistry usually receive serum. They test the serum for different components.
- Immunology test for antibodies.
- Serology receive serum samples to look for evidence

of diseases such as hepatitis or HIV.

— Histology process solid tissue removed from the body to make slides and examine cellular detail.

— Cytology examine smears of cells (such as from the cervix) for evidence of cancer and other conditions.

— Cytogenetics involves using blood and other cells to get a karyotype. This can be helpful in prenatal diagnosis (e.g. Down's syndrome) as well as in cancer (some cancers have abnormal chromosomes).

— Virology and DNA analysis are also done in large medical laboratories.

Sample Processing

Sample processing will usually start with a set of samples and a request form.

Typically a set of vacutainer tubes containing blood, or any other specimen will arrive to the laboratory in a small plastic bag, along with the form.

The form and the specimens are given a laboratory number. The specimens will usually all receive the same number, often as a sticker that can be placed on the tubes and form. Entry of requests onto a laboratory management system involves typing, or scanning (where barcodes are used) in the laboratory number, and entering the patient identification, as well as any tests requested. This allows laboratory machines, computers and staff to know what tests are pending, and also gives a place (such as a hospital department, doctor or other customer) for results to go.

For biochemistry samples, blood is usually centrifuged and serum is separated. If the serum needs to go on more than one machine, it can be divided into separate tubes.

Many specimens end up in one or more sophisticated automated analyser, that process a fraction of the sample and return one or more "results".

Laboratory Informatics

Laboratories today are held toghether by a system of software programmes and computers that exchange data about patients, test requests and test results, known as Laboratory information system.

This system enables hospitals and labs to send the correct test requests for each sample and keep track of individual patient or sample history, and help to guarantee a better quality of results, as well as publishing the results for doctors to check and patients to read.

Case study: The Work of a General Hospital Laboratory

The work which may be undertaken by the laboratory of a General Hospital can be classified as follows:

1. *From Hospital In patients:* This is similar to the work done in any public hospital in New Zealand, for all laboratory facilities must be available to the sick soldier. In addition there will be extra bacteriological and transfusion work from battle casualties and work related to the tropical or other diseases endemic and epidemic to the area. Details are given below.
2. *From Hospital Outpatients:* A base hospital often made its specialists available in outpatient clinics to the units encamped in the neighbourhood and some work from this source fell to the laboratory.
3. *From the 'Area':* This would include water and milk analyses from camps in the area; investigation of outbreaks of food poisoning; material from RAPs

and station sick quarters; the doing of serological tests from VD treatment centres, etc.

4. *Transfusion Work:* It was found better to have the servicing of apparatus, preparation of solutions and maintenance of the blood bank under care of the laboratory; in some hospitals the Pathologist bled the donors and supervised actual transfusions.
5. *Research Work:* An enormous amount of material from the sick, from battle casualties, and from epidemics was received by laboratories: there is considerable opportunity for research which may produce valuable results—but adequate staff is essential.

Types of Laboratory

In many countries, there are two main types of labs that process the majority of medical specimens. Hospital laboratories are attached to a hospital, and perform tests on these patients. Private (or community) laboratories receive samples from general practitioners, insurance companies, and other health clinics for analysis.

For extremely specialised tests, samples may go to an environmental science or research laboratory.

A lot of samples are sent between different labs for uncommon tests. It is more cost effective if a particular laboratory specialises in a rare test, receiving specimens (and money) from other labs, while sending away tests it cannot do.

Analysis of Work Done at 1 NZ General Hospital Laboratory During Thirty-One Months at Helwan

This analysis is based on the monthly reports furnished to the Deputy Director of Pathology, Middle East, and is set out in full month by month in the following table. The graph shows the fluctuation of work, relating it to the monthly admissions.

Following is the total of specimens examined in thirty-one months under the various headings in the monthly reports:

Specimens Examined

Enteric group fevers	3613
Dysentery	9113
Helminthiasis	396
Malaria	5906
Other protozoology	7
Relapsing fever	128
Undulant fever	42
Typhus fever	25
Throat swabs	2927
Sputa	2329
Pus, skin scales, etc.	814
Wound infections	678
Venereal disease	10353
Biochemistry	1865
Vaccines made	139
Blood counts	11169
Puncture fluids	739
Urines	5919
Food, milk, water	355
Histological sections	569
Post-mortems	139
Blood-grouping	725
Grand total	57,950

Consideration of the above figures shows:

1. That the average number of specimens examined per month fell little short of 2000. The average

figure for Christchurch Hospital over a two-year period (1948–50) was approximately 3000.The staff at 1 NZ General Hospital was 5 technicians, most of whom were partly trained; the staff at Christchurch Hospital during the above period was 17, trained or in training.

2. That about one-third of the work done arose from tropical diseases.
3. Work arising from battle casualties made only a small contribution (about 6 per cent) to the total (wound infections, part of blood counts and blood grouping).
4. A relatively small amount of biochemical work. Nevertheless, a wide range of chemical work was undertaken to provide all the tests normally available in a public hospital. This branch of the work is certain to show a large increase in any future war, and will require the services of a properly trained biochemist.
5. A high figure for tests under venereal disease: this was largely due to the laboratory undertaking serological tests for VD Treatment Centres in a large area.

The Central Pathology Laboratory

The RAMC Laboratory was attached to 15 Scottish Hospital in Cairo, and was under the supervision of the DDP ME and his staff. It was used as a reference laboratory on many subjects. In particular it carried out Wassermann tests checking our positive Kahn tests, investigated anaerobic bacteria, phage-typed strains of typhoid bacilli.

The DDP ME paid regular and most helpful visits to the laboratories under his command and held an annual conference of pathologists at which current problems were discussed, recent advances in technique described, and papers on research projects presented.

Through the DDP it was arranged for the reference to any one pathologist of all the material arising from certain diseases so that sufficient material for research could be assembled.

Analysis of Post-mortem Examinations Made at 1 General Hospital, Helwan, October 1941 to March 1944

Admissions—

Surgical (incl over 2000 battle casualties)		10,500 approx
Medical		15,000 approx
Total (includes other than New Zealanders)		25,500
Deaths	91	
Post-mortems carried out—		
On hospital deaths	90	
'Brought in dead'	43	
	133	

Causes of Death in Hospital—

Battle casualties	21
Pneumococcal infections	11
Following accidents	10
Following burns	6
Staphylococcal infections	6
Tuberculosis	4
Infective hepatitis	4
Typhoid fever	4
Typhus fever	3
Diphtheria	3

Malaria	1
Miscellaneous	18
	91

Causes of Death of Soldiers 'Brought in Dead'

Murder	1
Suicide	8
Accident (vehicle and falls)	21
GSW (accidental)	3
Drowning	1
Natural causes	9
	43

Epidemic and Endemic Diseases

Enteric Fever: Cases of enteric fevers occurred occasionally, but there was one outbreak in the latter half of 1943 which involved much laboratory work—in one month 762 specimens (blood cultures, urines, and faeces) were derived from this source alone, 'clearance' specimens contributing largely to the total.

Dysentery: Bacillary and amoebic dysentery were endemic—peak months were November 1941, October 1942, and September 1943, when 358, 732, and 662 specimens of faeces were respectively examined. Careful search for amoebae in every case of dysentery throws much work on the laboratory staff.

Malaria: This too was endemic, but showed peak months which unfortunately almost coincided with the peak dysentery months—September 1942, 428; August 1943, 567 specimens examined.

Infective Hepatitis: Many cases were admitted during the Middle East epidemics—few were fatal. The laboratory work involved consisted of blood counts, icterus indices, and urine and faeces for bile pigments. While much of this work was not essential it was felt important to take advantage of the epidemics to make some laboratory studies. Much more might have been done with adequate staff.

Diphtheria: Occasional cases occurred throughout the period. At the end of 1942 there was both an increase in faucial diphtheria and in diphtheritic infection of wounds. At one stage the nursing staff were Schick tested and the susceptible members immunised.

Number Required

Consideration of the volume of work done (as shown above) indicates that the technical staff necessary in a General Hospital laboratory is at least:

1. Technician-in-Charge: This man should be properly qualified and experienced.
2. Technician for general bacteriology.
3. Technician for faeces and urine examinations.
4. Technician for biochemistry—a properly trained biochemist.
5. Technician for media making and section cutting.
6. Technician for haematology.
7. 'Trainee' or general duties man for washing up, sterilising, etc.
8. Spare Technician: At base hospitals each man was entitled to 1½ days off duty per week and to two annual leave periods of 14 days; as a technician cannot be replaced by a general duties man a 'spare' is an essential.

9. Transfusion Orderly, if blood transfusion work and intravenous solution preparation is undertaken by the laboratory.

This suggested staff of 8 (plus transfusion orderly = 9) for dealing with approximately 2000 specimens per month may be contrasted with the Christchurch Hospital staff of 17 (plus 3 transfusion staff=20) for dealing with approximately 3000 specimens per month.

In 1940 the first General Hospitals went to the Middle East with each a Pathologist and each *one* partly trained technician (private). It was soon found that the RAMC War Establishment provided for 600 and 900-bed hospitals laboratory assistants as follows:

Sergeant technician	1
Private technician	1

and this establishment appears to have been that of 2 NZEF in 1942, as under the capitation agreement with the British Government the 2 NZEF WE was tied to the British. The difficulty of staff shortage in laboratories was overcome by 'attaching' nursing orderlies (privates) 'for training'. Thus in August 1943, 1 NZ General Hospital (average daily bed state over 800) had three 'attached for training' and a 'transfusion orderly'. Even this staff necessitated much 'overtime' and night work in the many busy periods.

This 'attachment for training' was later prohibited, resulting in a report to DMS by the Pathologist 1 NZ General Hospital (October 1943) indicating the work undertaken and staff required much as above, and suggesting an establishment of:

	600 Beds	*900 Beds*	*1200 Beds*
Sergeant	1	1	1
Technicians	3	5	6

(exclusive of orderlies for transfusion work and for 'area work' if undertaken).

In November 1943 the War Establishment was amended to:

	600 Beds	*900 Beds*
Sergeant	1	1
Corporal	1	1
Privates	2	3

which was a step in the right direction.

Rank of Laboratory Technicians

Shortly after the amendment to the 2 NZEF WE in November 1943 it was found that the WE for 3 Division in the Pacific was:

General Hospital	(600 beds):
Staff-Sergeant	1
Sergeants	3
WAAC	2

The 2 NZEF WE compared very unfavourably with this, and it seemed that the technicians who had served long and worked hard in the Middle East had been treated unjustly in contrast. Accordingly it was suggested that after:

— 3 months a trainee should become Lance-Corporal
— 9 months a trainee should become Corporal
— 18 months a trainee should become Sergeant

if there was a vacancy for a sergeant on the establishment.

In reply it was suggested from the office of the DGMS that qualified technicians on enlistment should become sergeants at once and that trainees 'after 6 months efficient service' should become sergeants. The first of these proposals was fair: the second over generous.

However, it was recognised as a bad principle that the different divisions of the New Zealand Army should have different ranks for personnel doing the same work—and letters to this effect reached the Minister of Defence and appeared in the daily papers. One difficulty lay in the question of similar rank for radiographers, dispensers, etc.

Finally, after considerable correspondence in July 1944, the WE for 2 NZEF was amended to:

	General	*Hospitals*
	600 beds	*900 beds*
Staff-Sergeant	1	1
Sergeant	1	1
Corporal	1	2
Lance-Corporal	2	2

For the future it might be suggested that the Senior Technician-in-charge should be a qualified and experienced 'Hospital Bacteriologist' and should be given commissioned rank. There should also be in every General Hospital laboratory a technician with considerable experience in biochemistry.

A General Hospital laboratory should always have a Pathologist (Medical Officer) in charge.

General Hospital Laboratory Equipment

The laboratories of the General Hospitals in 2 NZEF were in the main furnished with standard RAMC equipment.

This was well thought out and of good quality. It was designed to operate anywhere, and as kerosene was the fuel for incubators, sterilisers, etc., it was independent of electric light and gas, though when available these were, of course, used for heating and lighting. With the standard equipment, and using its boxes as benches and cupboards, it was possible to operate an efficient laboratory in a hospital tent, as, for example, 1 NZ General Hospital laboratory at Farsala in Greece. Criticism may be made of the rather cumbrous design of some of the larger laboratory pieces—e.g., the incubators, which could be better designed for transport. Other suggestions for improvement are:-

1. Provision of at least four microscopes for a hospital of 600 beds.
2. Provision of some sort of microscope lamp (? high-pressure mantle type, kerosene burning) for use when electricity is not available.
3. Provision of a better centrifuge (electric or hand).
4. Provision of better haematological apparatus-Haemoglobinometer, better quality counting chambers and pipettes.
5. Provision of a colorimeter (the MRC Grey Wedge Photometer could well be used) for biochemistry—this would enable the more usual standard biochemical methods to be used.

On a future occasion it might well be ascertained in advance what sort of laboratory equipment a General Hospital might expect at its destination overseas.

Training of Technicians

The first two General Hospitals reached the Middle East with each a single technician—partly trained in one case and slightly trained in the other—a fantastically inadequate provision, when it is known how much work fell on the hospital laboratories.

Not until 1943 was any attempt made to provide trained technicians from New Zealand (and then these were sent with rank already above those who had trained and worked long in the Middle East).

Training of technicians was therefore carried out in all the General Hospital laboratories and proved very satisfactory. It must, however, be emphasized that a trainee is for a considerable time of no use—in fact, an encumbrance—in a laboratory, and that a nucleus of several trained (qualified) technicians is essential for the provision of a first-class laboratory service.

HOSPITAL CASE MANAGEMENT

Hospital case management is a collaborative process that assesses, plans, implements, coordinates, monitors and evaluates the options and services required to meet an individual's health needs, using communication and available resources to promote quality, cost-effective outcomes in the hospital environment.

A hospital case manager coordinates the clinical goals with the patient's goals and manages the financial and quality outcomes of the care provided. With appropriate training, education and direction, hospital case managers can use their skills to affect a balanced clinical and financial outcome.

HOSPITAL AUTHORITY

The Hospital Authority is a statutorybody managing all the public hospitals and institutes. It is managed by the Hospital Authority Board and is under the monitor of the Secretary for Health and Welfare of the HKSAR Government.

History

Before the establishment of the authority, all health and medical issues were under the management of he Medical and Health Department. In 1990, a new health administration system was introduced. The department became the Department of Health and in 1991, the management of all the public hospitals was passed to a new statutory body, the Hospital Authority, which was established in 1990 under the Hospital Authority Ordinance. In 2003, the General Outpatient Clinics of Department of Health were transferred to the Authority.

MEDICAL TECHNOLOGY

Meducak technology refers to the diagnostic or therapeutic application of science and technology to improve the management of health conditions. Technologies may encompass any means of identifying the nature of conditions and intervening with devices, pharmacological, biological or other methods to increase life span and/or improve the quality of life.

Medical Technology or MedTech for short may refer to a college degree or course where a graduate becomes a Medical Technologist by profession or RMT (Registered Medical Technologist). Medical Technology is often referred as clinical laboratory science. This type of profession usually involves working in an a hospital analyzing laboratory specimens such as blood, semen, and other human secretions. Medical Technology is often taken as a pre-medical course, since its curriculum is very helpful for students who intend on taking up medicine as a profession and/or becoming a doctor.

HEALTHCARE TERMINOLOGIES AND CLASSIFICATION SYSTEMS

The terms disease and remedy were formerly understood and therefore defined quite differently to what they are now; so, likewise, are the meanings and definitions of inflammation, pneumonia, typhus, gout, lithiasis, &c., different from those which were attached to them thirty years ago...It is evident ... that great mischief will in most cases ensue if, in such attempts at definition and explanation, greater importance is attached to a clear and determinate, than to a complete and comprehensive understanding of the objects and questions before us. In a field like ours, clearness can in general be purchased only at the expense of completeness and therefore truth.

Oesterlen, Medical Logic, (1855)

Coding and classification systems have a long history in medicine. Current systems can trace their origins back to epidemiological lists of the causes of death from the early part of the eighteenth century. François Bossier de Lacroix (1706-1777) is commonly credited with the first attempt to classify diseases systematically (ICD-10, 1993). Better known as Sauvages, he published the work under the title *Nosologia Methodica.*

Linnaeus (1707-1778) who was a contemporary of Sauvages also published his Genera Morborum in that period. By the beginning of the nineteenth century, the Synopsis Nosologiae Methodicae, published in 1785 by William Cullen of Edinburgh (1710-1790) was the classification in most common use.

It was John Graunt who, working about a hundred years earlier, is credited with the first practical attempts to classify disease for statistical purposes. Working on his

London Bills of Mortality, he was able to estimate the proportion of deaths in different age groups. For example, he estimated a 36% mortality for liveborn children before the age of 6. He did this by taking all the deaths classified as convulsions, rickets, teeth and worms, thrush, abortives, chrysomes, infants, and livergrown. To these he added half of the deaths classed as smallpox, swinepox, measles, and worms without convulsions. By all accounts his estimate was a good one (ICD-10, 1993).

It has only been in the last few decades that these terminological systems have started to attract wide-spread attention and resources. The ever growing need to amass and analyse clinical data, no longer just for epidemiological purposes, has provided considerable incentive and resources for their development. Further, with the development of computer technology, there has been a belief that such wide-spread collection and analysis of data are now possible. In parallel, the requirement for clinicians to participate in that data collection has meant that they have had more opportunity to work with terminologies, and begin to understand their benefits and limitations.

In the basic concepts of term, code, and classification were introduced. In this chapter, several of the major coding and classification systems in routine use in healthcare will be introduced, and their features compared. Some specific limitations of each system will be highlighted. In reality there are a large number of such systems in development and use, and they cannot all be identified here. The systems discussed are however representative of most systems in common use, and can serve as an introduction to them. Throughout, a historical perspective will be retained, since in this case the lessons of the past have deep implications for the present. The more general limitations of all terminological systems will be addressed.

The International Classification of Diseases

Purpose. The International Classification of Diseases (ICD) is published by the World Health Organisation (WHO). Currently in its tenth revision (ICD-10), its goal is to allow morbidity and mortality data from different countries around the world to be systematically collected and statistically analysed. It is not intended, nor is it suitable, for indexing distinct clinical entities (Gersenovic, 1995). The International Nomenclature of Diseases (IND) provides the set of recommended terms and synonyms that correspond to the entries classified in the ICD codes.

History. The ICD can trace its ancestry to the early days of healthcare terminologies. William Farr (1807-1883) became the first medical statistician for the General Register Office of England and Wales. Upon taking office, he found the Cullen classification in use, but that it had not been updated in accordance with medical advances, nor did it seem suitable for statistical purposes. In his first Annual Report of the Registrar General, he noted:

> 'The advantages of a uniform statistical nomenclature, however imperfect, are so obvious, that it is surprising that no attention has been paid to its enforcement in Bills of Mortality. Each disease has, in many instances, been denoted by three or four terms, and each term has been applied to as many different diseases: vague, inconvenient names have been employed, or complications have been registered instead of primary diseases. The nomenclature is of as much importance in this department of enquiry as weights and measures in the physical sciences, and should be settled without delay. (ICD-10, 1993).'

Farr toiled hard at improving the classification, and by 1855, the International Statistical Congress adopted a classification based on the work of Farr, and Marc d'Espine of Geneva. Subsequently steered by Jaques Bertillon, this developed into the International List of Causes of Death. This was adopted in 1893, and continued to develop through the turn of the century and beyond, and ultimately evolved into the current ICD system.

In particular, the system was expanded to include not just causes of death, but diseases resulting in measurable morbidity. This expansion started with the urging of Farr. It was supported by Florence Nightingale, who in 1860 urged the adoption of Farr's disease classification for the tabulation of hospital morbidity in her paper Proposals for a uniform plan of hospital statistics. In 1900 at the First International Conference to revise the Bertillon Classification, a parallel classification of diseases for use in statistics of sickness was finally adopted.

Level of acceptance and use. The ICD today is used internationally by WHO for comparison of statistical returns. It is also adopted by many individual countries in the preparation of their statistical returns. Most other major classification systems endeavour to make their systems compatible with ICD, so that data coded in these systems can be mapped directly to ICD codes. ICD thus acts as a defacto reference point for many healthcare terminologies.

Classification structure. The ICD-10 is a multiple-axis classification system. At its core, the basic ICD is a single list of three alphanumeric character codes. These are organised by category, from A00 to Z99 (excluding U codes which are reserved for research, and for the provisional assignment of new diseases of uncertain aetiology). This level of detail is the mandatory level for reporting to the WHO mortality database and for general international comparisons.

2

List of Hospital Departments

- Anatomy
- Anaesthesiology
- Ayurvedic medicine
- Biochemistry and Clinical Nutrition
- Blood bank
- Cardiology
- Cardiovascular and Thoracic Surgery
- Chest Medicine and Environment Pollution Research Center (EPRC)
- Clinical Pharmacology
- Dentistry
- Diamond Jubilee Society Trust
- Ear, Nose and Throat Surgery
- Emergency Medical Services
- Endocrinology
- Forensic Medicine and Toxicology
- Gastroenterology
- General Surgery
- GSMC-FAIMER Regional Institute
- Hematology

— Library
— Medical Education Technoloy Cell
— Medicine
— Microbiology
— Neonatology
— Nephrology
— Neurology
— Neurosurgery
— Nursing
— Obstetrics & Gynecology
— Occupational Therapy
— Ophthalmology
— Orthopedics
— Pathology
— Pediatric Surgery
— Pediatrics
— Pharmacology
— Physiology
— Physiotherapy School & Center
— Plastic Surgery
— Preventive and Social Medicine
— Psychiatry
— Radiology
— Sexually Transmitted Diseases and Skin
— Social Service
— Surgical Gastroenterology
— Urology

3

Select List of Hospitals in India

Delhi

— AIIMS, Ansari Nagar
— Apollo Hospital, Sarita Vihar
— Batra Hospital, Hamdard Nagar
— Safdarjung Hospital
— Escorts Heart Institute, Okhla
— Fortis Health Care Limited, Delhi
— Modi Hospital, Saket
— Holy Family Hospital, Vasant Vihar
— Ganga Ram Hospital, Rajendar Nagar
— Max Devki Devi Heart and Vascular Institute, Saket
— Max Medcentre, Panchsheel Park
— Max Hospital, Pitampura
— Max Hospital, Noida
— Max Balaji Hospital, Patparganj
— Lady Hardinge, Punchkuian Road
— MAMC, Delhi Gate
— Venu Eye Institute, Sheikh Sarai
— Ram Manohar Lohia Hospital, Wellingdon Crescent
— G.B. Pant Hospital
— National Heart Institute, East of Kailash
— Lok Nayak Jaiprakash Narain Hospital, Jawahar Lal Marg

— St. Stephens Hospital, Civil Lines
— Moolchand Medcity, Lajpat Nagar III, New Delhi 110 024
— Bara Hindu Rao Hospital, Sabzi Mandi
— Deen Dayal Upadhyay Hospital, Hari Nagar
— E.S.I. Hospital, Jhilmil Area
— Jaipur Golden Hospital, Rohini
— Jankidas Kapur Memorial Hospital, Naraina Road
— Kolmet Hospital & Medical Research Centre, Pusa road
— Maharaja Agarsain Hospital, Ashok Vihar
— Natinal Health Institute, East of Kailash
— Ram Manohar Lohia Hospital,, Kharag Singh Marg
— Shri Ram Heart Institute & Reseach Centre, Kirti Nagar
— Sitaram Bharita Institute, Qutab Institutional Area
— Vasant Lok Hospital, Vasant Vihar
— Vardaan Hospital, Malviya Nagar

Mumbai

— Bhatia Hospital, Tardeo
— Bhabha Hospital, Chembur
— Bombay Hospital
— Breach Candy
— Cooper Hospital
— Goculdas Tejpal Hospital
— Grant Medical College and Sir Jamshedjee Jeejebhoy Group of Hospitals
— Hinduja Hospital, Mahim
— Holy Family Hospital, Bandra
— Holy Spirit Hospital, Andheri
— Hurkisondas Hospital, Girgaum
— Jeevan Hospital, Malad

— Karuna Hospital, Borivali
— KEM Hospital, Parel
— Leelavati Hospital, Bandra
— Lokmanya Tilak Hospital, Sion
— Nair Hospital, Bombay Central
— Rajawadi Hospital, Ghatkopar
— Saifee Hospital
— S.K. Patil Arogyadham, Malad
— Shroff Eye Hospital, Bandra - accredited by Joint Commission International
— St George Hospital, CST
— Tata Memorial Hospital
— Wockhardt Hospital, Mulund - accredited by Joint Commission International

Chennai

— Madras Medical Mission
— Sri Ramachandra Medical College and Research Institute
— Sri Ramachandra Dental College
— CSI Kalyani Multi-Speciality Hospital
— Dr. Mehta's Hospital Private Limited
— Dr. Mehta's Multi-Speciality
— Vijaya Hospital
— Apollo Hospital
— Billroth Hospital
— Malar Hospitals
— Kaliappa Hospital
— Frontier lifeline hospital
— Apollo first med
— Apollo speciality hospital for women
— Lifeline hospital
— Govt general hospital

— Stanley medical college hospital
— Kilpauk medical college hospital
— Srm hospital
— Hande hospitals
— Govt royapettah hospital
— Kanchi children's hospital
— M.V. diabetes centre
— Sankara nethralaya
— MIOT hospitals
— Railway hospital
— Trinity hospital
— Harvey heart hospital
— Hindu mission hospital
— Rigid hospital
— SMF hospital and research centre
— zubeida hospital
— Rex hospitals
— Child trust hospital
— Esi hospital
— Kumaran hospital
— Adyar cancer research institute

Kolkata

— Calcutta Medical College
— Apollo Hospital
— Westbank Hospital
— NRS Medical Hospital
— Calcutta National Medical College
— Calcutta Medical Reaearch Institute
— AMRI
— Peerless Hospital
— Furkan Hospital
— Daisy Memorial Mental Hospital

Kerala

— Arobana Hospital (Thodupuzha) Idukki
— Assisi Skin Clinic (Thodupuzha) Idukki
— S.H. Medical Center Kottayam
— Bharath Hospital Kottayam
— Medical College Kottayam
— Karipal Hospital Kottayam
— Amala Cancer Hospital and Research Center Thrissur
— Medical Trust Hospital Pathanamthitta
— Amrita Institute of Medical Science & Research Centre, Ernakulam
— Lakeshore Hospital & Research Centre Ltd., Cochin
— Aswini Hospital Thrissur
— Medical College Thrissur
— Mannarkkad Nursing Home,Palakkad
— Moonniyoor nursing Home (Chemmad) Malappuram
— Tirurangadi Nursing Home (Chemmad) Malappuram
— Al-Shifa Hospital (Perinthalmanna) Malappuram
— Kerala Institute of Medical Science, Trivandrum
— Sree Chitra Thirunal Institute of Medical Sciences and Technology, Trivandrum
— Regional Cancer Centre (RCC), Trivandrum
— Cosmopolitan Hospitals, Trivandrum
— Medical College Hospitals, Trivandrum
— Sri Avittom Thirunal Hospital for Women and Children (SAT), Trivandrum
— Gokulam Medical College Hospital, Venjarammood, Trivandrum
— Homeopathic Medical College Hospital, Trivandrum
— Ayurvedic Medical College Hospital, Trivandrum
— St. Thomas Hospital (Chethipuzha) Kottayam
— P.V.S. Memorial Hospital (Kaloor) Ernakulam
— Lissy Hospital (Kaloor) Ernakulam

- Medical Trust Ernakulam Medical Trust Ernakulam
- Little Flower Hospital Angamali and Research Center
- Cheriyapally Hospital Kottayam
- Bhavana Hospital Kottayam

Jharkhand

- Tata Main Hospital, Jamshedpur
- Tinplate Hospital, Jamshedpur
- RIMS, Ranchi
- Bokaro General Hospital, Bokaro Steel Plant,Steel Authority of India Limited, Bokaro.

Hyderabad

- Care Hospital, Banjara Hills
- Usha Mullapudi Cardiac centre, Jeedimetla
- Osmania General Hospital
- St. Theresa's Hospital, Erragadda
- Nature Cure Hospital, Balkampet

Bangalore

- Bangalore Medical College, K.R. Road
- Victoria Hospital (Bangalore Medical College)
- Vanivilas Women and childrens hospital, Bangalore Medical College
- Bowring & Lady Curzon Hospitals, Bangalore Medical College
- Minto eye hospital, Bangalore Medical College
- SDS T.B sanitorium, Bangalore Medical College
- St. Johns Medical College
- Wockhardt Hospital, Cunningham Rd.
- Kempegowda Institute of Medical Sciences, K.R. Road
- M.S. Ramaiah Hospital
- Dr. B.R. Ambedkar Hospital
- Sri Rajarajeshwari Medical College and Hospital, Mysore road

- Vydehi Institute of Medical Sciences
- Manipal Hospital, Airport Road
- Mallya Hospital
- Narayana Hrudayalaya, Hosur Road
- Narayana Nethralaya, Chord Road
- Netradhama, Kanakapura Road
- St. Marthas Hospital, Nrupatunga Road
- National Institute of Mental Health and Neuro Sciences(NIMHANS)
- Kidwai Memorial Institute of Oncology
- Sri Jayadeva Institute of Cardiology
- Nethradhama Superspeciality Eye Hospital, Jayanagar

Others (Arbitrarily Selected)

- Sankara Eye Hospital, Coimbatore
- Sankara Eye Hospital, Guntur
- Sankara Rural Eye Hospital, Krishnankovil
- Chaithanya Eye Hospital, Thiruvananthapuram
- Indus Hospital, Shimla
- Medical Trust Hospital, Cochin - general surgery
- MCV Memorial ENT Trust Hospital, Coimbatore - endoscopic sinus, micro ear, laryngeal, head, and neck surgery
- Specialists' Hospital, Cochin - plastic and microvascular surgery, urodynamics, ophthalmology, cardiology, physiatry, orthopedics
- Vega ENT Hospital, Coimbatore - ear, nose, and throat disorders
- CMC, Vellore
- narayan hrudayalaya, Blore
- Vaatsalya Hospital Gadag, Hubli, Karwar

4

Select List of Hospitals Worldwide

LIST OF HOSPITALS IN ALABAMA

— Andalusia Regional Hospital – Andalusia, Alabama
— Athens-Limestone Hospital – Athens, Alabama
— Atmore Community Hospital – Atmore, Alabama
— Baptist Cherokee – Centre, Alabama
— Baptist Citizens – Talladega, Alabama
— Baptist DeKalb – Fort Payne, Alabama
— Baptist Lawrence – Moulton, Alabama
— Baptist Medical Center East – Montgomery, Alabama
— Baptist Medical Center South – Montgomery, Alabama
— Baptist Montclair – Birmingham, Alabama
— Baptist Princeton – Birmingham, Alabama
— Brookwood Medical Center – Birmingham, Alabama
— Bryce State Mental Hospital – Tuscaloosa, Alabama
— Carraway Methodist Hospital – Birmingham, Alabama
— Children's Hospital of Alabama – Birmingham, Alabama
— Crestwood Medical Center – Huntsville, Alabama
— Cullman Regional Medical Center – Cullman, Alabama
— Decatur General Hospital System – Decatur, Alabama
— East Alabama Medical Center – Opelika, Alabama

— Eye Foundation Hospital – Birmingham, Alabama
— Fayette Medical Center – Fayette, Alabama
— Flowers Hospital – Dothan, Alabama
— Gadsden Regional Medical Center – Gadsden, Alabama
— Hartselle Medical Center – Hartselle, Alabama
— Helen Keller Hospital – Sheffield, Alabama
— Huntsville Hospital System – Huntsville, Alabama
— Infirmary Medical Center – Mobile, Alabama
— Infirmary West at Knollwood – Mobile, Alabama
— Jackson Hospital and Clinic – Montgomery, Alabama
— Lanier Health Services – Valley, Alabama
— Marshall Medical Center North – Guntersville, Alabama
— Marshall Medical Center South – Boaz, Alabama
— Medical Center Enterprise – Enterprise, Alabama
— Monroe County Hospital – Monroeville, Alabama
— Parkway Medical Center – Decatur, Alabama
— Providence Hospital – Mobile, Alabama
— Riverview Regional Medical Center – Gadsden, Alabama
— Russell Medical Center – Alexander City, Alabama
— Southeast Alabama Medical Center – Dothan, Alabama
— Springhill Memorial Hospital – Mobile, Alabama
— St. Vincent's Hospital – Birmingham, Alabama
— UAB Hospital – Birmingham, Alabama
— University of South Alabama Medical Center – Mobile, Alabama
— University of South Alabama Children's and Women's Hospital – Mobile, Alabama
— Veterans Administration Hospital – Birmingham, Alabama
— Woodland Medical Center – Cullman, Alabama

LIST OF HOSPITALS IN ALASKA

— Alaska Native Medical Center (Anchorage)
— Alaska Regional Hospital (Anchorage)
— Bartlett Regional Hospital (Juneau)
— Central Peninsula General Hospital (Soldotna)
— Ketchikan General Hospital (Ketchikan)
— Mat-Su Regional Medical Center (Palmer)
— Petersburg Medical Center (Petersburg)
— Providence Alaska Medical Center (Anchorage)
— Providence Kodiak Island Medical Center (Kodiak)
— Sitka Community Hospital (Sitka)
— South Peninsula Hospital (Homer)
— Wrangell Medical Center (Wrangell)

LIST OF HOSPITALS IN ARKANSAS

— Arkansas Children's Hospital - Little Rock, Arkansas
— Arkansas Heart Hospital - Little Rock, Arkansas
— Arkansas Methodist Hospital - Paragould, Arkansas
— Baptist Health Medical Center Arkadelphia - Arkadelphia, Arkansas
— Baptist Health Medical Center Heber Springs - Heber Springs, Arkansas
— Baptist Health Medical Center Little Rock - Little Rock, Arkansas
— Baptist Health Medical Center North Little Rock - North Little Rock, Arkansas
— Baxter Regional Medical Center - Mountain Home, Arkansas
— Carroll Regional Medical Center - Berryville, Arkansas
— Conway Regional Health System - Conway, Arkansas
— Summit Medical Center - Van Buren, Arkansas
— Crittenden Memorial - West Memphis, Arkansas

— Drew Memorial Hospital - Monticello, Arkansas
— Hot Spring County Medical Center - Malvern, Arkansas
— Jefferson Regional Medical Center - Pine Bluff, Arkansas
— Johnson Regional Medical Center - Clarksville, Arkansas
— Levi Hospital - Hot Springs, Arkansas
— Medical Center of South Arkansas - El Dorado, Arkansas
— Medical Park Hospital - Hope, Arkansas
— Mena Medical Center - Mena, Arkansas
— National Park Medical Center - Hot Springs, Arkansas
— North Arkansas Regional Medical Center - Harrison, Arkansas
— Northwest Medical Center - London, Arkansas
— Ouachita County Medical Center - Camden, Arkansas
— Pinnacle Pointe Hospital - Little Rock, Arkansas
— Rebsamen Regional Medical Center - Jacksonville, Arkansas
— NEA Medical Center - Jonesboro, Arkansas
— St Bernards Behavioural Health - Jonesboro, Arkansas
— Saline Memorial Hospital - Benton, Arkansas
— St. Anthony's Healthcare Center - Morrilton, Arkansas
— St. Edward Mercy Medical Center - Fort Smith, Arkansas
— St. Joseph's Mercy Health Center- Hot Springs, Arkansas
— St. Mary's Hospital - Rogers, Arkansas
— Saint Mary's Regional Medical Center - Russellville, Arkansas
— St. Vincent Doctors Hospital - Little Rock, Arkansas
— St. Vincent Medical Center North - Sherwood, Arkansas
— Southwest Regional Medical Center - Little Rock, Arkansas

- Sparks Regional Medical Center - Fort Smith, Arkansas
- Stuttgart Regional Medical Center - Stuttgart, Arkansas
- UAMS Medical Center, the hospital of the University of Arkansas for Medical Sciences - Little Rock, Arkansas
- Washington Regional Medical Center - Fayetteville, Arkansas
- White County Medical Center - Searcy, Arkansas
- White River Medical Center - Batesville, Arkansas

LIST OF HOSPITALS IN ARGENTINA

City of Buenos Aires

- ALPI, Instituto de Rehabilitación "Marcelo Fitte"
- CEMIC, Av. Las Heras 2900
- CEMIC, Galván 4102
- FLENI, Fundación Lucha Contra Enfermedades Neurológicas Infantiles
- FUNDALEU, Fundación Argentina Contra la Leucemia
- Hospital Aeronático Central
- Hospital Militar Central
- Hospital Naval "Dr. Pedro Mallo"
- Complejo Médico Policial "Churruca-Visca"
- Hospital de Clínicas "José de San Martín" (UBA)
- Hospital Odontológico Universitario (UBA)
- Hospital General de Agudos "Donación Francisco Santojanni", Mataderos
- Hospital Municipal de Oncología "Marie Curie", Agronomía
- Hospital de Niños "Pedro Elizalde"
- Hospital "Manuel Belgrano"
- Hospital Alemán
- Hospital Español
- Hospital Centro Gallego de Buenos Aires

— Hospital Infanto Juvenil "C. Tobar García", Barracas
— Hospital Nacional de Pediatría "Profesor Dr. Juan P. Garrahan", Constitución
— Hospital Italiano de Buenos Aires
— Hospital Francés
— Hospital Británico
— Hospital Israelita - ISRAMED
— Hospital y Administración Nacional de Laboratorios e Institutos de Salud "Dr. Carlos G. Malbrán", ANLIS
— Hospital de Infecciosas "Dr. Francisco Muñiz", Parque Patricios
— Hospital General de Agudos "D. Vélez Sarsfield", Liniers
— Hospital de Emergencias Psiquiátricas "Torcuato de Alvear", Agronomía
— Hospital Odontológico (ex Nacional), Recoleta
— Hospital de Odontología "José Dueñas", Almagro
— Hospital de Odontología Infantil "Don Benito Quinquela Martín", La Boca
— Hospital Municipal de Rehabilitación Psicofísica, I.R.E.P. , Nuñez
— Hospital de Gastroenterología "B. Udaondo", Barracas
— Hospital General de Agudos "Cosme Argerich", La Boca
— Hospital Neuropsiquiátrico de Varones "J. T. Borda", Barracas
— Hospital General de Agudos "Dr. Carlos G. Durand", Caballito
— Hospital "Dr. Juan A. Fernández"
— Hospital de Niños "Ricardo Gutiérrez", Palermo
— Hospital General de Niños "Pedro de Elizalde", Constitución
— Hospital de Rehabilitación Respiratoria "María Ferrer"
— Hospital General de Agudos "Dr. Ignacio Pirovano", Coghland

— Hospital Municipal de Quemados, Caballito
— Hospital General de Agudos "Dr. J. M. Ramos Mejía", Balvanera
— Hospital Materno Infantil "Ramón Sardá", Parque Patricios
— Hospital Nacional "Bernardino Rivadavia", Recoleta
— Hospital Oftalmológico "Dr. Pedro Lagleyze", Villa Gral. Mitre
— Hospital Municipal de Oftalmología "Santa Lucía", San Cristóbal
— Hospital General de Agudos "Dr. Enrique Tornú", Villa Ortúzar
— Hospital de Rehabilitación Respiratoria "M. Ferrer", Barracas
— Hospital de Salud Mental de Mujeres "Braulio Moyano", Barracas
— Hospital General de Agudos "Dr. Abel Zubizarreta", Villa Devoto
— Hospital General de Agudos "Dr. T. Alvarez" , Flores
— Hospital General de Agudos "J. A. Penna", Parque Patricios
— Hospital General de Agudos "P. Piñero", Flores
— Instituto de Zoonosis "Luis Pasteur", Caballito
— Instituto de Rehabilitación Psicofísica "M. Rocca", Flores
— Instituto de Cardiología y Cirugía Cardiovascular "F. Favaloro"
— Instituo Dupuytren de Traumatología y Ortopedia
— I.N.C.U.C.A.I.
— Instituto de Investigaciones Médicas "Alfredo Lanari" (UBA)
— Instituto de Oncología "Angel Roffo" (UBA)
— Instituto de Tisioneumología "Raúl F. Vacarezza" (UBA)
— Servicio Nacional de Rehabilitación

Province of Buenos Aires

— H. Municipal General "Anita Ellicagaray, A. Gonzáles Cháves
— H. Interzonal General de Agudos "Dr. J. Penna", Bahía Blanca
— H. Municipal "Dr. L. Lucero", Bahía Blanca
— H. Menor "Ing. White", Ingeniero White
— H. Municipal de Agudos "María Eva Duarte de Perón"
— H. Municipal, Oriente
— H. Municipal "Dr. Cabrera", Coronel Pringles
— H. Municipal "Eva Perón", Punta Alta
— H. Municipal, Coronel Suárez
— H. Municipal "Lucero del Alba", Huanguelén
— H. Municipal "Dr. Joaquín Llambías", Guaminí
— H. Menor "Dr. Ramón Carrillo", Monte Hermoso
— H. Municipal de Agudos "Dr. Pedro Ecay", Carmen de Patagones
— H. Municipal, Villalonga
— H. Municipal "Gobernador Ugarte", Puán
— H. Municipal "Villa Iris", Villa Iris
— H. Local "General San Martín", Carhué
— H. de Ancianos "General N. Levalle", Carhué
— H. "Dr. Noé Yarcho", Rivera
— H. "Demetrio carmelo Layarte", Villa Mazza
— Hospital Nacional de Lepra "Dr. Baldomero Sommer", RP 24, 3.5 km RN 6, Partido General Rodríguez
— Hospital Nacional de Agudos "Profesor Dr. Alejandro Posadas", El Palomar
— Instituto Nacional de Enfermedades Virales Humanas "Dr. Julio I. Maiztegui", INEVH, Pergamino
— Hospital Regional de Agudos "San José", Pergamino
— Hospital Regional de Agudos "San Felipe", San Nicolás de los Arroyos

— Hospital "Virgen del Carmen" - Zárate http://www.ms.gba.gov.ar/imagenes/Guia_2005.pdf

Hospitales Gran Buenos Aires Norte

— H. Municipal "Dr. Bernardo Houssay, Vicente López
— H. Zonal de Agudos y Crónicos "Dr. Cetrángolo, Vicente López
— H. de Niños Municipal "San Isidro", San Isidro
— H. Municipal de San Isidro, San Isidro
— H. Zonal General de Agudos "M. V. de Martínez", Tigre
— H. Zonal General de Agudos "Petrona V. de Cordero", San Fernando
— H. Municipal Dr. D. E. Thompson, San Martín
— H. Interzonal General de Agudos "Eva Perón" (ex Castex), San Martín
— H Zonal de Agudos "Gral. Manuel Belgrano", San Martín
— H. Municipal "Dr. R. Larcade", San Miguel
— Clínica Independencia, Munro
— Clínica Olivos, Olivos
— Sanatorio "San Lucas", San Isidro
— H. Materno Infantil "San Isidro", San Isidro
— Hospital Juan C. Sanguinetti, Pilar (Víctor Vergani 860)

Hospitales de Gran Buenos Aires Oeste

— H. Zonal General de Agudos "Prof. Dr. Ramón Carrillo", Ciudadela
— H. Interzonal General de Agudos "Dr. L. Güemes", Haedo
— Posadas
— H. Zonal General de Agudos "Dr. Diego Paroissien", Isidro Casanova

— H. "San Juan de Dios", Ramos Mejía
— Clínica Güemes, Luján
— Clínica Modelo Morón, Morón
— H. Virtual de Morón

Hospitales de Gran Buenos Aires Sur

— H. Interzonal General de Agudos "Evita", Lanús
— H. Interzonal General de Agudos "Dr. Pedro Fiorito", Avellaneda
— H. Interzonal General de Agudos "Pte. Perón", Sarandí
— H. Zonal General de Agudos "Dr. Isidoro Iriarte, Quilmes
— H. Interzonal General de Agudos "L.C. de Gandulfo", Lomas de Zamora
— H. Zonal General de Agudos "Lucio Meléndez", Adrogué
— H. Interzonal General de Agudos "J. A. Estévez", Temperley
— H. Municipal "Mi Pueblo", Florencio Varela
— H. Zonal General de Agudos Descentralizado "Evita Pueblo", Berazategui
— H. Zonal de Agudos Ezeiza, Ezeiza
— Clínica Modelo de Lanús, Lanús
— Policlínico UOM, Avellaneda
— Clínica Sanatorio "Modelo", Quilmes Oeste

Hospitales City of La Plata

— H. Interzonal General de Agudos "General San Martín"
— H. Interzonal General de Agudos "Prof. Dr. R. Rossi"
— H. Zonal General de Agudos "Dr R. Gutiérrez"
— H. Zonal General de Agudos "San Roque", Manuel B. Gonnet
— H. Interzonal General de Agudos y Crónicos "San Juan de Dios"
— H. Interzonal General de Agudos "Sor María Ludovica"

— H. Español "de La Plata"
— H. Italiano "de La Plata"

Province of Catamarca

— H. Provincial José Chain, Andalgalá
— H. Regional Belén, Belén
— H. Zonal de Icaño, Icaño
— H. "Roberto Ramón Carrillo", Pomán
— H. San José, Santa María
— H. Área Nº 3 "La Merced", La Merced
— H. Distrital Villa D, Las Tejas De Valle Viejo
— H. "El Rodeo", El Rodeo
— H. R. R. Carro, Chumbicha
— H. "San José, Piedra Blanca
— H. Zonal de Recreo, Recreo
— H. "Dr. Liborio Forte", Recreo
— H. Distrital de Saujil, Saujil
— H. Zonal "San Juan Bautista", Tinogasta

City of Catamarca

— H. Interzonal "San Juan Bautista"
— H. Centro de Rehabilitación
— H. Centro de Salud
— H. Interzonal de Niños

Province of Córdoba

— H. Vecinal Achiras, Achiras
— H. Vecinal Adelia María, Adelia María
— H. Municipal Alcira, Alcira
— H. de Beneficencia, Alejandro
— H. Vecinal, Alejandro
— H. M. Salvador Esca, Almafuerte
— H. Arturo Humberto, Alta Gracia
— Policlínico Ferroviario, Alta Gracia

— H. de Arias, Arias
— H. Municipal "Dr. Carlos Julio Rodríguez", Arroyito
— Complejo Asistencial Regional, Bell Ville
— H. Municipal, Buchardo
— H. Vecinal, Camilo Aldao
— H. Cañada De Luque, Cañada de Luque
— H. Municipal "San José", Canals
— H. "San Antonio de Padua", Río Cuarto

City of Córdoba, Argentina

— H. Aeronáutico Cordoba
— H. Amelia S L de
— H. Español
— H. Gustavo A
— H. Hernan
— H. Italiano
— H. José
— H. Mediterráneo Central
— H. Militar Cordoba
— Policlínico Policial
— H. Privado Sa
— H. Roberto J
— H. Sagrado Corazón De Jesús
— Instituto Del Quemado
— H. Aeronáutico, Av. Colón 479
— H. Aeronáutico, Av. F Aérea Arg km 6,5
— H. Córdoba
— H. de Niños
— H. de Pediatría
— H. de Urgencias
— H. Infantil Municipal
— H. Materno Provincial
— H. Misericordia, Pje Caeiro 1259

- H. Misericordia, Belgrano 1502
- H. Misericordia, Ayacucho 1700
- H. Neuropsiquiátrico
- H. Rawson
- H. San Roque
- H. T. C. de Allende
- H. Universitario de Mat Y N
- Policlínico Ferroviario

Province of Corrientes

City of Corrientes

- H. "Ángela I. de Llano"
- H. Escuela "General San Martín"
- H. de Niños
- H. Psiquiátrico
- H. Geriátrico
- Instituto de Cardiología

Province of Formosa

City of Formosa

- H. Central
- H. de "La Madre y el Niño"

Province of Misiones

- H. de Área Apóstoles, Apóstoles

Province of Chaco

City of Resistencia

- H. "Perrando"
- H. "4 de Junio", Sáenz Peña

Province of Santa Cruz

- H. Regional Río Gallegos - Río Gallegos

Province of Santa Fe

— H. Escuela Eva Perón, Granadero Baigorria
— H. "San Carlos", Casilda
— H. "Anselmo Gamen", Villa Gobernador Gálvez
— H. "San José", Cañada de Gómez
— H. Central, Reconquista
— H. "A. Gutiérrez", Venado Tuerto

Rosario

— Centro Regional de Salud Mental Dr. Agudo Ávila
— H. de Niños Zona Norte
— H. Geriátrico Provincial
— H. Municipal Intendente Carrasco
— Hospital Provincial de Rosario
— Hospital Provincial del Centenario
— H. Italiano Giuseppe Garibaldi de Rosario
— H. Municipal Juan B. Alberdi
— Sanatorio Británico
— H. Español de Rosario
— H. Unione e Benevolenza
— H. de Niños Víctor J. Vilela
— H. "Roque Sáenz Peña"
— H. de Emergencias Clemente Álvarez (HECA)

San Lorenzo

— H. Granaderos a Caballo

Province of Tucumán

— H. Aguilares, Aguilares
— H. de Concepción, Aguilares
— H. Regional Concepción, Concepción
— H. Privado SRL, Concepción

— H. Belascuain, Concepción
— H. Bella Vista, Bella Vista
— H. "Gómez Llueca, Simoca
— H. "Gral. Lamadrid" , Monteros
— H. "Juan Bautista Alberdi", Juan Bautista Alberdi
— H. "Gral. Lamadrid ", Graneros
— H. "Los Sarmientos", Los Sarmientos
— H. "Mario Stivala", La Cocha
— H. Parajón Ortiz, Famailla
— H. "Santa Ana", Santa Ana
— H. Tafí del Valle, Tafí Del Valle
— H. Trancas, Trancas
— H. Avellaneda, Las Talitas
— H. "Ramón Humberto, Lamadrid

City of Tucumán

— H. Ángel C. Padilla
— H. Centro de Salud "Zenón Sant"
— H. "del Niño Jesús"
— H. "Juan Obarrio"
— H. "Nicolás Avellaneda"
— H. Privado de Flebología
— H. Privado de Ojos
— H. Psiquiátrico "del Carmen"
— H. de Niños Soc. Arg. de Pediatría

LIST OF HOSPITALS IN BANGLADESH

— Bangladesh Institute of Research and Rehabilitation for Diabetes, Endocrine and Metabolic Disorders (BIRDEM)
— Chittagong Maa-Shishu O General Hospital,Agrabad, Chittagong.
— Dhaka Hospital,Dhaka

— Apollo Hospitals, Dhaka (website)
— Dhaka Medical College Hospital.
— PG Hospital, Dhaka.
— Red Crescent Holy Famiy Hospital, Dhaka.
— Sir Salimullah Medical College Hospital, Dhaka.
— Chittagong Medical College Hospital.
— Rajshahi Medical College Hospital.
— Rangpur Medical College Hospital.
— Sylhet Medical College Hospital.
— Barisal Medical College Hospital.
— Mymensingh Medical College Hospital.
— CMH (Combined Military Hospital).
— BDR (Bangladesh Rifles) Hospital
— Bangladesh Medical College Hospital, Dhaka
— Central Hospital
— Basundhura Hospital (Pvt.) Ltd.
— Gonoshastaya Nagar Hospital
— Rashmono General Hospital
— Samorita Hospital Ltd.
— Z.H. Sikder Women's Medical Collage & Hospital (Pvt.) Ltd.
— Continental Hospital Ltd
— Anwer Khan Modern Hospital Ltd.
— Ibne Sina Hospital
— Apollo Hospital
— Medinova Hospital

LIST OF HOSPITALS IN CANADA

Alberta

— Banff
  - Banff Mineral Springs Hospital
— Barrhead
  - Barrhead Healthcare Centre

— Bassano
  - Bassano Health Centre
— Black Diamond
  - Oilfields General Hospital
— Blairmore
  - Crowsnest Pass Hospital
— Bow Island
  - Bow Island Health Centre
— Boyle
  - Boyle Healthcare Centre
— Brooks
  - Brooks Health Centre
— Calgary
  - Foothills Medical Centre
  - Alberta Children's Hospital
  - Peter Lougheed Centre
  - Rockyview General Hospital
— Camrose
- St. Mary's Hospital
— Canmore
  - Canmore Hospital
— Cardston
  - Cardston Hospital
— Castor
  - Our Lady of the Rosary Hospital
— Claresholm
  - Claresholm General Hospital
— Coronation
  - Coronation Hospital and Care Centre
— Daysland
  - Daysland Health Centre

— Devon
  - Devon General Hospital
— Drayton Valley
  - Drayton Valley Hospital and Care Centre
— Drumheller
  - Drumheller Health Centre
— Edmonton
  - Alberta Hospital Edmonton
  - Devon General Hospital
  - Grey Nuns Community Hospital & Health Centre
  - Leduc Community Hospital & Health Centre
  - Misericordia Community Hospital
  - Royal Alexandra Hospital
  - St Joseph's Auxiliary Hospital
  - Stollery Children's Hospital
  - Stony Plain Municipal Hospital
  - Sturgeon Community Hospital & Health Center
  - University Of Alberta Hospital
— Edson
  - Edson & District Healthcare Centre
— Fort Saskatchewan
  - Fort Saskatchewan General Hospital
— Grande Prairie
  - Queen Elizabeth II Hospital
— Hanna
  - Hanna Health Centre
— High Prairie
  - High Prairie Health Complex
— High River
  - High River General Hospital

— Hinton
 - Hinton General Hospital
— Innisfail
 - Innisfail Health Centre
— Lacombe
 - Lacombe Hospital and Care Centre
— Leduc
 - Leduc Community Hospital
— Lethbridge
 - Lethbridge Regional Hospital
— Lloydminster
 - Lloydminster Hospital
— Mayerthorpe
 - Mayerthorpe Healthcare Centre
— McLennan
 - Sacred Heart Community Health Centre
— Medicine Hat
 - Medicine Regional Hospital
— Milk River
 - Milk River Hospital
— Olds
 - Olds Hospital and Care Centre
— Oyen
 - Big Country Health Centre
— Peace River
 - Peace River Community Health Centre
— Pincher Creek
 - Pincher Creek Hospital
— Ponoka
 - Alberta Hospital Ponoka
 - Ponoka Hospital and Care Centre

— Raymond
  - Raymond Hospital
— Red Deer
  - Red Deer Regional Hospital and Care Centre
— Rimbey
  - Rimbey Hospital and Care Centre
— Rocky Mountain House
  - Rocky Mountain House Hospital and Care Centre
— Smoky Lake
  - George McDougall Health Centre
— St. Paul
  - St. Paul Health Care Centre
— Stettler
  - Stettler Hospital and Care Centre
— Strathmore
  - Strathmore District Health Services
— Sundre
  - Sundre Hospital and Care Centre
— Taber
  - Taber Hospital
— Three Hills
  - Three Hills Health Centre
— Trochu
  - St. Mary's Health Centre
— Vegreville
  - St. Joseph's General Hospital
— Vermilion
  - Vermilion Health Centre
— Vulcan
  - Vulcan Community Health Centre
— Wainwright
  - Wainwright Health Centre

— Wetaskiwin
  - Wetaskiwin Hospital and Care Centre

British Columbia

— Abbotsford
  - Menno Hospital
  - MSA Hospital

— Alert Bay
  - Cormorant Island Community Health Centre

— Ashcroft
  - Ashcroft and District Hospital

— Bella Coola
  - Bella Coola General Hospital

— Burnaby
  - Burnaby Hospital
  - Fellburn Hospital
  - St. Michael's Centre Extended Care Hospital

— Burns Lake
  - Lakes District Hospital and Health Centre

— Campbell River
  - Campbell River & District General Hospital

— Castlegar
  - Castlegar and District Community Health Centre

— Chemainus
  - Chemainus Health Care Centre

— Chetwynd
  - Chetwynd General Hospital

— Chilliwack
  - Chilliwack General Hospital

— Clearwater
- Dr. Helmcken Memorial Hospital

— Comox
- St. Joseph's Hospital

— Coquitlam
- Riverview Hospital

— Cranbrook
- East Kootenay Regional Hospital

— Creston
- Creston Valley Hospital

— Dawson Creek
- Dawson Creek and District Hospital

— Delta
- Delta Hospital

— Duncan
- Cowichan District Hospital

— Fernie
- Fernie District Hospital

— Fort Nelson
- Fort Nelson General Hospital

— Fort St. James
- Stuart Lake General Hospital

— Fort St. John
- Fort St. John General Hospital
- Peace Lutheran Extended Care Centre

— Golden
- Golden and District General Hospital

— Grand Forks
- Boundary Hospital

— Halzelton
- Wrinch Memorial Hospital

— Hope
  - Fraser Canyon Hospital
— Invermere
  - Invermere and District Hospital
— Kamloops
  - Overlander Extended Care Hospital
  - Royal Inland Hospital
— Kalso
  - Victorian Community Health Centre of Kaslo
— Kelowna
  - Kelowna General Hospital
— Kitimat
  - Kitimat General Hospital
— Ladysmith
  - Ladysmith and District General Hospital
— Langley
  - Langley Memorial Hospital
— Lytton
  - St Bartholomew's Hospital
— MacKenzie
  - Mackenzie and District Hospital
— Maple Ridge
  - Ridge Meadows Hospital & Health Care Centre
— Masset
  - Queen Charlotte Islands General Hospital – Masset Site
— McBride
  - McBride and District Hospital
— Merritt
  - Nicola Valley Health Centre
— Mission
  - Mission Memorial Hospital

— Nakusp
  - Mission Memorial Hospital Arrow Lakes Hospital
— Nanaimo
  - Nanaimo Regional General Hospital
— Nelson
  - Kootenay Lake Hospital
  - Mount St. Francis Hospital
— New Denver
  - Slocan Community Health Centre
— New Westminster
  - Queen's Park Hospital
  - Royal Columbian Hospital
— North Vancouver
  - Lions Gate Hospital
— Oliver
  - South Okanagan General Hospital
— 100 Mile House
  - 100 Mile District General Hospital
— Parksville
  - Trillium Lodge
— Penticton
  - Penticton Regional Hospital
— Port Alberni
  - West Coast General Hospital
— Port Alice
  - Port Alice Hospital
— Port Hardy
  - Port Hardy Hospital
— Port McNeill
  - Port McNeill and District Hospital
— Port Moody
  - Eagle Ridge Hospital & Health Care Centre

— Pouce Coupe
  - Pouce Coupe Care Home
— Powell River
  - Powell River General Hospital
— Prince George
  - Prince George Regional Hospital
— Prince Rupert
  - Prince Rupert Regional Hospital
— Princeton
  - Princeton General Hospital
— Qualicum Beach
  - Eagle Park Health Care Facility
— Queen Charlote City
  - Queen Charlotte Islands General Hospital
— Quesnel
  - G.R. Baker Memorial Hospital
— Revelstoke
  - Queen Victoria Hospital
— Richmond
  - The Richmond Hospital
— Saanichton
  - Saanich Peninsula Hospital
— Salmon Arm
  - Shuswap Lake General Hospital
— Salt Spring Island
  - The Lady Minto Gulf Islands Hospital
— Sechelt
  - St. Mary's Hospital
— Smithers
  - Bulkley Valley District Hospital
— Sparwood
  - Sparwood Health Centre

— Squamish
  - Squamish General Hospital
— Stewart
  - Stewart Health Centre
— Summerland
  - Summerland Health Centre
— Surrey
  - Surrey Memorial Hospital
— Terrace
  - Terrace Mills Memorial Hospital
— Tofino
  - Tofino General Hospital
— Trail
  - Kootenay Boundary Regional Hospital
— Vancouver
  - British Columbia Cancer Agency
  - British Columbia Children's Hospital
  - British Columbia Women's Hospital and Health Centre
  - Braddan Private Hospital
  - Brock Fahrni Pavilion
  - George Pearson Centre
  - G.F. Strong Centre
  - Holy Family Hospital
  - Kensington Private Hospital
  - Louis Brier Hospital
  - Mount Saint Joseph Hospital
  - Normandy Hospital
  - St. Paul's Hospital
  - St. Vincent's Hospital
  - Shriners Hospitals for Children
  - Sunny Hill Health Centre for Children

- Vancouver Hospital & Health Sciences Centre
  - § U.B.C. Health Sciences Centre Hospital
  - § Vancouver General Hospital

— Vanderhoof
- St. John Hospital

— Vernon
- Vernon Jubilee Hospital

— Victoria
- Juan de Fuca Hospitals
- Queen Alexandra Centre for Children's Health
- Royal Jubilee Hospital
- The Gorge Road Hospital
- Victoria General Hospital

— Waglisla
- R.W. Large Memorial Hospital

— White Rock
- Peace Arch Hospital

— Williams Lake
- Cariboo Memorial Hospital

[edit] Manitoba

— Thompson
- Thompson General Hospital

— Selkirk
- Selkirk & District General Hospital

— Winnipeg
- Concordia Hospital
- Grace General Hospital
- Health Sciences Centre
- Misericordia General Hospital
- Saint Boniface General Hospital
- Seven Oaks General Hospital

- Victoria General Hospital
- Winnipeg Children's Hospital

New Brunswick

— Government of New Brunswick - List of regional services by Health Region

— Bathurst
  - Chaleur Regional Hospital/Hôpital régional Chaleur

— Cambellton
  - Campbellton Regional Hospital

— Edmundston
  - Edmundston Regional Hospital

— Fredericton
  - Dr. Everett Chalmers Regional Hospital

— Grand Manam
  - Grand Manan Hospital

— Lamèque
  - Hôpital et Centre de santé communautaire de Lamèque

— Miramichi
  - Region 7 Hospital

— Moncton
  - Hôpital régional Dr-George-L.-Dumont
  - Moncton Hospital

— Sackville
  - Sackville Memorial Hospital

— Sainte-Anne-de-Kent
  - Hôpital Stella-Maris-de-Kent H

— Saint John
  - Saint John Regional Hospital
  - St. Joseph's Hospital

- St. Stephen
  - Charlotte County Hospital
- Sussex
  - Sussex Health Centre
- Tracadie-Sheila
  - Hôpital de Tracadie-Sheila
- Waterville
  - Upper River Valley Hospital-opening in 2006
- Woodstock
  - Carleton Memorial Hospital

Newfoundland and Labrador

Government of Newfoundland and Labrador - List of regional services by Health Region

- Baie Verte
  - Baie Verte Peninsula Health Centre
- Bonavista
  - Bonavista Peninsula Health Centre
- Bonne Bay
  - Bonne Bay Health Centre
- Botwood
  - Dr. Hugh Twomey Health Centre
- Brookfield
  - Brookfield Bonnews Health Care Centre
- Buchans
  - A.M Guy Memorial Health Centre
- Burgeo
  - Calder Health Centre
- Burin
  - Burin Peninsula Health Care Centre

— Carbonear
  - Carbonear General Hospital
— Charlottetown
  - Charlottetown Community Clinic
— Clarenville
  - Dr. G.B. Cross Memorial Hospital
— Corner Brook
  - Dr. J. I. O'Connell Centre
  - Western Memorial Regional Hospital
— Flower's Cove
  - Strait of Belle Isle Health Centre
— Fogo
  - Fogo Island Hospital
— Forteau
  - Labrador South Health Centre
— Gander
  - James Paton Memorial Hospital
— Gaultois
  - Gaultois Clinic
— Grand Bank
  - Grand Bank Community Health Centre
— Grand Falls-Windsor
  - Central Newfoundland Regional Health Centre
— Green Bay
  - Green Bay Community Health Centre
— Happy Valley-Goose Bay
  - Labrador Health Centre
— Harbour Breton
  - Connaigre Peninsula Community Health Centre
— Harbour Deep
  - Harbour Deep Community Clinic

— Hermitage
  - Hermitage Clinic
— La Scie
  - La Scie Medical Centre
— Labrador City
  - Captain William Jackman Memorial Hospital
— Lewisporte
  - Lewisporte Lab & X-Ray Clinic
— Mary's Harbour
  - Mary's Harbour Community Clinic
— McCallum
  - McCallum Visiting Clinic
— Milltown
  - Bay D'Espoir Medical Clinic
— Mount Carmel
  - Mount Carmel Medical Clinic
— Old Perlican
  - Dr. A.A. Wilkinson Memorial Health Centre
— Placentia
  - Placentia Health Centre
— Port aux Basques
  - Dr. Charles L. Legrow Health Centre
— Port Hope Simpson
  - Port Hope Simpson Community Clinic
— Port Saunders
  - Rufus Guinchard Health Centre
— Rencontre East
  - Mose Ambrose Clinic
  - Rencontre Clinic
— Roddickton
  - White Bay Central Health Centre

— St. Anthony
  - Dr. Charles S. Curtis Memorial Hospital
— St. John's
  - Dr. Leonard A. Miller Centre
  - Dr. Walter Templeman Health Centre
  - General Hospital, Health Sciences Centre
  - Janeway Children's Health and Rehabilitation Centre
  - St. Clare's Mercy Hospital
  - Waterford Hospital
— St. Lawrence
  - U.S. Memorial Health Centre
— St. Lewis
  - St. Lewis Community Clinic
— St. Mary's Bay
  - St. Mary's Bay Medical Clinic
— Stephenville
  - Sir Thomas Roddick Hospital
— Twillingate
  - Notre Dame Bay Memorial Health Care Centre
— Whitbourne
  - Dr. W.H. Newhook Community Health Centre

Northwest Territories

— Fort Simpson
  - Fort Simpson Hospital
— Fort Smith
  - Fort Smith Health Centre
— Hay River
  - H.H. Williams Memorial Hospital
— Inuvik
  - Inuvik Regional Hospital

- Yellowknife
  - Stanton Regional Hospital

Nova Scotia

- Amherst
  - Highland View Regional Hospital / Cumberland Regional Health Care Centre
- Antigonish
  - St. Martha's Regional Hospital
- Bridgewater
  - South Shore Regional Hospital
- Digby
  - Digby General Hospital
- Halifax Regional Municipality
  - Dartmouth
    - § Dartmouth General Hospital
    - § Nova Scotia Hospital
    - § East Coast Forensic Hospital
  - Halifax Peninsula
    - § IWK Health Centre
    - § Queen Elizabeth II Health Sciences Centre
  - Lower Sackville
    - § Cobequid Community Health Centre
  - Middle Musquodoboit
    - § Musquodoboit Valley Memorial Hospital
  - Musquodoboit Harbour
    - § Twin Oaks Memorial Hospital
  - Sheet Harbour
    - § Eastern Shore Memorial Hospital
- Inverness
  - Inverness Consolidated Memorial Hospital
- Kentville
  - Valley Regional Hospital

— Liverpool
  - Queens General Hospital
— Middleton
  - Soldiers Memorial Hospital
— New Glasgow, Nova Scotia
  - Aberdeen Hospital
— Shelburne
  - Roseway Hospital
— Sydney
  - Cape Breton Regional Hospital
— Truro
  - Colchester Hospital
— Yarmouth
  - Yarmouth Regional Hospital

Nunavut

— Iqaluit
  - Baffin Regional Hospital

Ontario

— Ajax
  - Ajax Pickering General Hospital
  - Rouge Valley Ajax Pickering
— Alliston
  - Stevenson Memorial Hospital
— Atikokan
  - Atikokan General Hospital
— Bancroft
  - North Hastings District Hospital
— Barrie
  - Royal Victoria Hospital
— Barry's Bay
  - St. Francis Memorial Hospital

— Bowmanville
  - Bowmanvill Memorial Hospital
— Bracebridge
  - South Muskoka Memorial Hospital
— Brampton
  - Brampton Civic Hospital
  - Brampton Memorial Hospital Campus
— Brockville
  - Brockville General Hospital
— Burlington
  - Joseph Brant Memorial Hospital
— Carleton Place
  - Carlton Place & District Memorial Hospital
— Chatham
- Public General Hospital
— Cobourg
  - Northumberland Hills Hospital
— Collingwood
  - Collingwood General And Marine Hospital
— Cornwall
  - Community Hospital McConnell Site
— Dunnville
  - Haldimand War Memorial Hospital
— Durham
  - Durham Memorial Hospital
— Englehart
  - Englehart and District Hospital
— Espanola
  - Espanola General Hospital
— Fergus
  - Groves Memorial Community Hospital

— Georgetown
  - Georgetown Hospital
— Geraldton
  - Geraldton District Hospital
— Guelph
  - Guelph General Hospital
  - Homewood Health Centre
  - St. Joseph's Health Centre
— Hagersville
  - Hagersville West Haldimand General Hospital
— Haliburton
  - Haliburton Hospital
— Hamilton
  - Hamilton Health Sciences
    § Chedoke Hospital
    § Hamilton General Hospital
    § Henderson General Hospital
    § Juravinski Cancer Centre
    § McMaster Children's Hospital
    § McMaster University Medical Centre (affiliated with McMaster University)
  - St. Joseph's Hospital
  - St. Peter's Hospital
— Hanover
  - Hanover District Hospital
— Huntsville
  - Huntsville Memorial District Hospital
— Ingersoll
  - Alexandra Hospital
— Kenora
  - Lake Of The Woods District Hospital

- Kincardine
  - Kincardine South Bruce Grey Health Centre
- Kingston
  - Kingston General Hospital
  - Kingston Hôtel Dieu Hospital
- Kirkland Lake
  - Kirkland and District Hospital
- Kitchener
  - St Mary's General Hospital
  - Grand River Hospital
  - Freeport Hospital
- Manitoulin
  - Manitoulin Health Centre
- London
  - London Health Sciences Centre
    - § Children's Hospital of Western Ontario
    - § South Street Hospital
    - § University Hospital
    - § Victoria Hospital
  - St. Joseph's Health Care, London
    - § Parkwood Hospital
    - § St. Joseph's Hospital
- Manitouwadge
  - Manitouwadge General Hospital
- Marathon
  - Wilson Memorial Hospital
- Markdale
  - Centre Grey General Hospital
- Meaford
  - Meaford General Hospital

— Midland
  - Huronia District Hospital
— Milton
  - Milton District Hospital
— Mindemoya
  - Mindemoya Hospital
— Minden
  - Minden Hospital
— Mississauga
  - Credit Valley Hospital
  - Trillium Health Centre
— Moose Factory
  - Moose Factory Hospital
— Mount Forrest
  - Louise Marshall Hospital
— New Liskeard
  - Temiskaming Hospital
— Nipigon
  - Nipigon District Memorial Hospital
— Oakville
  - Oakville-Trafalgar Memorial Hospital
— Ottawa (see also: List of hospitals in Ottawa)
  - Children's Hospital of Eastern Ontario (CHEO)
  - Montfort Hospital
  - National Defence Medical Centre
  - The Ottawa Hospital (formerly: Riverside Hospital, General Hospital, Civic Hospital)
  - Queensway-Carleton Hospital
  - University of Ottawa Heart Institute
  - Royal Ottawa Hospital
— Owen Sound
  - Grey Bruce Health Services

- Palmerston
  - Palmerston & District Hospital
- Parry Sound
  - Parry Sound Ambulance Hospital
- Pembroke
  - Pembroke Regional Hospital
- Perth
  - Great War Memorial Hospital
- Peterborough
  - Peterborough Civic Hospital
- Port Colborne
  - Port Colborne General Hospital
- Port Perry
  - Community Memorial Hospital
- Red Lake
  - Margaret Cochenour Memorial Hospital
- Regional Municipality of Waterloo
  - Kitchener-Waterloo Hospital
- Renfrew, Eastern Townships
  - Renfrew Victoria Hospital
- Simcoe
  - Norfolk General Hospital
- Smiths Falls
  - Smith Falls Community Hospital
- St. Catharines
  - Hôtel Dieu Hospital
- Sturgeon Falls
  - West Nipissing General Hospital
- Sudbury
  - Hôpital Régional de Sudbury Regional Hospital
    - § Hôpital Régional de Sudbury Regional Hospital | Laurentian Site

§ Hôpital Régional de Sudbury Regional Hospital | Memorial Site

§ Hôpital Régional de Sudbury Regional Hospital | St. Joseph's Health Centre

- Sudbury Algoma Hospital

— Thunder Bay

- Thunder Bay Regional Health Science Centre

— Timmins

- Timmins & District Hospital

— Toronto (see also: List of hospitals in Toronto)

- Baycrest Centre for Geriatric Care
- Clarke Institute of Psychiatry
- Etobicoke General Hospital
- Hospital for Sick Children
- Humber River Regional Hospital
- Mount Sinai Hospital
- North York General Hospital
- North York General Hospital - Branson
- Queensway General Hospital
- Rouge Valley Centenary (Rouge Valley Regional Health Centre)
- Scarborough Hospital
- Scarborough Hospital - Grace
- St. Joseph's Health Centre
- St. Michael's Hospital
- Sunnybrook Health Sciences Centre
- Toronto East General Hospital
- Toronto Grace Hospital
- Toronto Rehab (Toronto Rehabilitation Institute)
- University Health Network

§ Princess Margaret Hospital

§ Toronto General Hospital

    - § Toronto Western Hospital
  - Women's College Hospital
- — Upsala
  - Ontario Ministry of Health
- — Uxbidge
  - Uxbidge Cottage Hospital
- — Walkerton
  - County of Bruce General Hospital
- — Welland
  - Welland County General Hospital
- — Woodstock
  - Woodstock General Hospital
- — York Region
  - Markham-Stouffville Hospital
  - York Central Hospital
  - Shouldice Hernia Centre
  - Southlake Regional Health Centre

Prince Edward Island

- — Alberton
  - Western Hospital
- — Charlottetown
  - Hillsborough Hospital
  - Queen Elizabeth Hospital, Prince Edward Island
- — Montague
  - Kings County Memorial Hospital
- — O'Leary
  - Community Hospital
- — Souris
  - Souris Hospital
- — Summerside
  - Prince County Hospital

— Tyne Valley
  - Stewart Memorial Hospital

Quebec

— *see also CLSC*
— Gatineau
  - Hôpital de Gatineau
— Laval
  - Cité de la Santé de Laval
  - Jewish Rehabilitation Hospital
— Montreal
  - Allan Memorial Institute
  - Douglas Hospital
  - Centre hospitalier de Fleury
  - Montreal Heart Institute
  - Hôpital Jean-Talon
  - Centre hospitalier de Lachine
  - Centre Hospitalier Pierre-Boucher
  - Lakeshore General Hospital
  - Centre hospitalier de LaSalle
  - Hôpital Louis-Hyppolite Lafontaine (Hôpital Louis-H. Lafontaine)
  - Hôpital Maisonneuve-Rosemont
  - McGill University Faculty of Medicine/MUHC
    § Montreal Chest Institute
    § Montreal Children's Hospital
    § Montreal General Hospital
    § Montreal Neurological Hospital
    § Royal Victoria Hospital
  - Centre hospitalier de Mont-Sinaï
  - Centre hospitalier Richardson
  - Hôpital Rivière-des-Prairies

- Hôpital du Sacré-Coeur de Montréal
- Centre hospitalier de St-Mary
- Hôpital Santa Cabrini
- Shriners Hospital-Canada
- Sir Mortimer B. Davis Jewish General Hospital
- Centre hospitalier universitaire de Montréal (affiliated to the Université de Montréal)
- Centre hospitalier universitaire Sainte-Justine (also affiliated to the Université de Montréal but independent from the Centre hospitalier universitaire de Montréal)
  - § Centre de réadaptation Marie-Enfant
- Centre hospitalier de Verdun

— Saint-Hyacinthe
- Centre hospitalier Honoré-Mercier

— Sherbrooke
- Centre hospitalier universitaire de Sherbrooke (CHUS)

Saskatchewan

— Assiniboia
- Assiniboia Union Hospital

— Balcarres
- Balcarres Hospital

— Big River
- Big River Hospital

— Broadview
- Broadview Union Hospital

— Canora
- Canora Hospital

— Carrot River
- Carrot River Union Hospital

— Cupar
  - Cupar Health Centre
— Davidson
  - Davidson Hospital
— Fillmore
  - Fillmore Health Centre
— Foam Lake
  - Foam Lake Health Centre
— Goodsoil
  - L. Gervais Memorial Hospital Centre
  - Kamsack, Saskatchewan | Kamsack Union Hospital
— Kerrobert
  - Kerrobert Hospital
— Kindersley
  - Kindersley Hospital
— La Rouge
  - La Ronge Health Centre
— Lanigan
  - Lanigan Hospital
— Loon Lake
  - Loon Lake Hospital
— Maidstone
  - Maidstone Hospital
— Maple Creek
  - Maple Creek Hospital
— Melfort
  - Melfort Hospital
— Moose Jaw
  - Moose Jaw Union Hospital
— Nipawin
  - Nipawin Hospital

— North Battleford
  - Battlefords Union Hospital
— Prince Albert
  - Victoria Hospital
— Regina
  - Regina General Hospital
  - Pasqua Hospital
— Saskatoon
  - Royal University Hospital
  - St. Paul's Hospital
— Swift Current
  - Swift Current Regional Hospital:

Yukon

— Whitehorse, Yukon
  - Whitehorse General Hospital
— Watson Lake, Yukon
  - Watson Lake Hospital

LIST OF HOSPITALS IN CHINA

— First Affiliated Hospital of Nanjing Medical University
— Jiangsu Provincial People's Hospital
— Jiangsu Provincial Traditional Chinese Medicine Hospital
— Jiangsu Provincial Stomatology Hospital
— Nanjing Union Dental Clinic
— Nanjing Gulou Hospital
— Nanjing Stomatology Hospital
— Nanjing Brain Hospital
— Nanjing Ophthalmology Hospital
— SOS International Clinic
— VIP Clinic of Jiangsu Province Hospital
— Suzhou Medical College Hospitals

LIST OF HOSPITALS IN EGYPT

This is a list of hospitals in Egypt:

Cairo

— Alexandria Psychiatric centre
— Agooza
— Ain Shams Specialized Hospital
— Al Salam
— Al Salam International
— Amoun Hospital
— Anglo-American
— Arab Contractors Medical Center
— Asyout University Hospital
— Badran
— Cairo Institute of Radiology
— Cairo Kindey Center
— Cleopatra
— Coptic
— Dar El Swefa Hospital
— Dar el Oyoun Hospital
— Demerdash
— El Fayrouz
— El Galaa
— El Gomhoureya
— El Kablat Hospital
— El Kateb Cairo
— El Madina Cairo
— El Merghany Hospital
— El Mobarra Maadi
— El Nozha International Hospital
— El Safa
— El Shark Hospital
— Garden City

— Hayat Medical Center
— Heliopolis Cardiac Center
— Ibn Sina
— Italian
— Misr International
— Nasser General
— New Kasr El Aini Hospital
— Red Crescent
— Roxy
— Shaalan Surgi Center
— The Universital Hussein

Alexandria

— Alex Radiology Center
— Alexandria Medical Center
— Armed Forces
— Coptic Hospital
— Dermatological
— Dr. Hassab
— Dr. Ibrahim Obeid
— Dr. Mohamed Milad
— Dr. Mohamed Nabawi El Mohandes
— Dr. Shalaby Alexandria
— El Amin El Kheireya Alexandria
— El Anba Takla Alexandria
— El Hadara University.
— El Kabbari
— El Madina El Tebbeya
— El Mowassah
— El Saghr Specialized
— El Seguini

— El Shatby Pediatric
— Fevers
— Gamal Abdel Nasser
— Main University Alexandria Koleyet
— Maternity Alexandria
— Miami Private
— Mohamed Ragab El Kheiry
— Sidi Bishr Alexandria El Sekka
— Victoria Hospital

Specialized Hospitals

Bone Diseases

— Helal Hospital - Specialized in bone surgery.

Pediatrics

— Abu El Reesh Hospital - The hospital is specialized in pediatrics, It was established with the collaboration of Japanese Government.

Heart Diseases

— Nasser Institute - Specialized in heart surgery.
— Embaba-Keet Kat
— Cairo Center for heart catheter (Cairo Cath).
— Heliopolis heart center - Heliopolois
— Dar el Fouad (Heart clinic and surgery)
— Alexandria center for heart catheter
— International heart center - Alexandria.

Kidney Diseases

— (Renal dialysis unit) centers

Renal dialysis units are existed in many specialized hospitals whether they belong to the universities or special ones Mansoura International Center for kidney diseases

International center for kidney diseases and renal diaysis in Egypt and the Middle East. It contains renal dialysis units and a specialized group of surgeons performing kidney surgery. The center is in the downtown in Mansoura.

— Kidney stones disintegration centers - ElKatteb Center
— El Salam Hospital (kidney center)
— The National Institute for kidney

Liver Diseases

— The National Institute for liver diseases (Menofya)

The institute is part of Menofya University. It is situated in Shebeen el Koum. Menofya-Shebeen el Koum.

— International Center for digestive system diseases
— Thudor Belharez Institute

Eye Diseases

— Eye diseases Institute Giza
— El Maghraby eye Center
— International eye center
— National Institute for eye diseases and surgery
— Suzan Mubarak Center for eye tumor (the first center in Arab area and North Africa)
— Mostafa Kamel Military Hospital - Alexandria.
— German Hospital - Alexandria.

Tumors

— National Tumor Institute

The Institute is attached to Kasser El Enie medical Hospital, specialized in treating tumors either by radiation or surgery.

— Syzium Center Kasser el Eini
— Egypt International center

Psychiatric

— Psychometrics - Behman Psychiatric Hospital
— Dr.Omar Shaheen Psychiatric Hospital
— Maadi Palace for Psychometrics

LIST OF HOSPITALS IN ENGLAND

London

North Central London

Name	*Locale*	*Opened*	*Closed*
Barnet General Hospital	Barnet		
Chase Farm Hospital	Enfield	1948	
Great Ormond Street Hospital for Sick Children	Bloomsbury	1852	
Hospital of St John and St Elizabeth	St John's Wood		
Middlesex Hospital	Middlesex		
North Middlesex Hospital	Edmonton		
Royal Free Hospital	Hampstead	1828	
University College Hospital	Euston	1834	
Whittington Hospital	Highgate	1848	

North East London

Name	*Locale*	*Opened*	*Closed*
Harold Wood Hospital	Harold Wood		
Homerton University Hospital	Homerton, London		
King George Hospital	London Borough of Redbridge		
London Lock Hospital	Hyde Park Corner, London	1747	1953
Moorfields Eye Hospital	London Borough of Islington	1805	
National Hospital for Neurology and Neurosurgery	Bloomsbury, London	1859	
Newham General Hospital	Plaistow	1983	
Oldchurch Hospital	Romford		
Queen's Hospital	Romford	17th December	2006

Rush Green Hospital	Rush Green	1900	1994
St Andrew's Hospital			
Royal London Hospital	Whitechapel, London	1785	
St Bartholomew's Hospital	Smithfield, London	1123	
St Clement's Hospital			
Wanstead Hospital	Wanstead	1938	1986
Whipps Cross University Hospital	Leytonstone		

North West London

- — Hammersmith Hospital
- — Central Middlesex Hospital, 243 beds
- — Chelsea and Westminster Hospital,
- — Ealing Hospital - Southall, Beds: 400
- — Harefield Hospital - Middlesex
- — Hillingdon Hospital - Hillingdon
- — Mount Vernon Hospital - Hillingdon
- — Northwick Park Hospital, Beds: 558
- — Royal National Orthopaedic Hospital - Stanmore, 220 Beds
- — St Mary's Hospital - Paddington
- — West Middlesex Hospital
- — Western Eye Hospital

South East London

Name	*Locale*	*Opened*	*Closed*
Beckenham Hospital	Beckenham		
Bethlem Royal Hospital	Beckenham	1330, 1930 at present site	
Evelina Children's Hospital	Lambeth	2005	
Greenwich Hospital	Greenwich		closed
Guy's Hospital	Southwark	1721	
King's College Hospital	Camberwell	1840, 1913 at present site	
Lambeth Hospital	Stockwell	1871 as South Western Hospital, early 1990s present name	
Lewisham Hospital	Lewisham		

Maudsley Hospital	Camberwell	1923
Mayday University Hospital	Thornton Heath	1885 as workhouse infirmary, 1866 present site, 1923 present name
Orpington Hospital	Orpington	
Princess Royal University Hospital	Orpington	
Queen Elizabeth Hospital	Woolwich	2001
St. Thomas' Hospital	Lambeth	described as 'ancient' in 1215, present site 1860s

South West London

— Chelsea & Westminster Hospital - Chelsea, (SW10)
— Cromwell Hospital, (SW5)
— Kingston Hospital – Kingston-upon-Thames
— Royal Brompton Hospital, Chelsea, (SW3)
— Royal Hospital Chelsea,(SW3)
— Royal Hospital for Neuro-disability - Putney, (SW15)
— St George's Hospital - Tooting, (SW17)
— St Mary Abbot's Hospital, Kensington, (W8 - closed)
— Royal Marsden Hospital, Chelsea, (SW3)
— Westminster Hospital, (SW1 - closed)

Other Strategic Health Authorities

East Midlands

— Derby City Hospital
— Derbyshire Royal Infirmary - Derby
— George Eliot Hospital - Nuneaton
— Glenfield General Hospital - Glenfield, Leicestershire
— Grantham & District Hospital - Grantham, Lincolnshire
— Kettering General Hospital - Kettering, Northamptonshire
— King's Mill Hospital - Sutton-in-Ashfield, Nottinghamshire
— Leicester General Hospital - Leicester

- Leicester Royal Infirmary - Leicester
- Nottingham City Hospital NHS Trust - Nottingham
- Queen's Medical Centre - Nottingham
- St Andrew's Hospital - Northampton charitable - UK's largest private hospital

East of England

- Addenbrooke's Hospital - Cambridge, 1,300 Beds
- Bedford Hospital - Bedford, 520 Beds
- Edith Cavell Hospital - Peterborough, Cambridgeshire
- Ipswich Hospital - Ipswich
- James Paget Hospital - Gorleston, Great Yarmouth, Norfolk
- Norfolk and Norwich University Hospital - Norwich
- Norwich Community Hospital - Norwich
- Papworth Hospital - Cambridgeshire
- Prestwich Hospital - Bury St Edmunds, Suffolk
- Queen Elizabeth Hospital, King's Lynn - King's Lynn, Norfolk
- Rampton Secure Hospital - Nottinghamshire
- Walnut Tree Hospital - Sudbury, Suffolk
- West Suffolk Hospital - Bury St Edmunds, Suffolk, 664 Beds

North East

- Bishop Auckland General Hospital - Bishop Auckland
- Chester-le-Street Hospital - Chester-le-Street
- Cleveland Nuffield Hospital - Stockton-on-Tees
- Darlington Memorial Hospital - Darlington
- Freeman Hospital - Newcastle
- Hexham General Hospital - Hexham
- The James Cook University Hospital - Middlesbrough

— Middleton St George Hospital - Middleton St George
— Newcastle General Hospital - Newcastle
— North Tyneside General Hospital - North Shields
— Royal Victoria Infirmary - Newcastle
— St Luke's Hospital - Middlesbrough
— St Nicholas Hospital - Gosforth
— University Hospital of North Durham - Durham
— University Hospital of Hartlepool - Hartlepool
— University Hospital of North Tees - Stockton-on-Tees
— Wansbeck General Hospital - Ashington
— West Lane Hospital - Middlesbrough

North West

— Ashworth Hospital
— Alder Hey Children's Hospital - Liverpool
— Altrincham General Hospital
— Birch Hill Hospital - Rochdale
— Blackpool Victoria Hospital - Blackpool, Lancashire
— Booth Hall Children's Hospital
— Broadgreen Hospital - Liverpool
— Carlisle Hospital - Carlisle
— Countess of Chester Hospital - Chester, Cheshire
— Fairfield Hospital - Bury
— Fazakerley Hospital - Liverpool
— Hope Hospital - Salford
— Leigh Infirmary - Leigh
— Macclesfield District Hospital - Macclesfield
— Manchester Royal Eye Hospital - Manchester
— Manchester Royal Infirmary - Manchester
— North Cheshire Hospital - Warrington
— North Manchester General Hospital
— Rochdale Infirmary
— Royal Albert Edward Infirmary - Wigan

- Royal Blackburn Hospital - Blackburn, opened on July 8th 2006 combines the two previous hospitals in Blackburn (Blackburn Royal Infirimiry and Queen's Park Hospital) into one main 'super-hospital', financed via the PFI
- Royal Bolton Hospital - Bolton
- Royal Liverpool Children's Hospital - Liverpool
- Royal Liverpool University Hospital - Liverpool
- Royal Manchester Children's Hospital - Pendlebury
- Royal Oldham Hospital - Oldham
- Royal Preston Hospital - Preston
- St Mary's Hospital for Women and Children - Manchester
- Stepping Hill Hospital - Stockport
- Tameside General Hospital - Ashton-under-Lyne
- Trafford General Hospital, Davyhulme, Manchester - formally Park Hospital- the first hospital in the NHS (1948)
- The Walton Centre for Neurology and Neurosurgery - Liverpool
- Warrington Hospital - Warrington
- Withington Hospital - Manchester
- Wythenshawe Hospital - Manchester

South East Coast

- Broadmoor Hospital
- Conquest Hospital - Hastings, East Sussex
- Eastbourne District General Hospital - Eastbourne, East Sussex
- Royal Sussex County Hospital - Brighton
- Royal Alexandra Hospital - Brighton
- Royal Surrey County Hospital - Guildford, Surrey
- Frimley Park Hospital - Aldershot, Surrey
- St Peter's Hospital - Chertsey, Surrey

— St Richard's Hospital - Chichester, West Sussex
— William Harvey Hospital - Ashford, Kent

South Central

— Royal Bournemouth Hospital - Bournemouth, Dorset
— Coldeast Hospital - Salisbury Green, Hampshire
— Gosport War Memorial Hospital - Gosport, Hampshire
— Havant War Memorial Hospital - Havant, Hampshire
— John Radcliffe Hospital – Oxford
— John Radcliffe Hospitals NHS Trust – Oxford, 1,500 Beds
— Lymington Hospital - Lymington
— Medway Maritime Hospital - Medway
— Moorgreen Hospital - West End, Hampshire
— Milton Keynes General Hospital - Milton Keynes - 460 Beds
— North Hampshire Hospital - Basingstoke
— Nuffield Orthopaedic Centre - Oxford
— Petersfield Hospital - Petersfield, Hampshire
— Poole Hospital - Poole, Dorset
— Queen Alexandra Hospital - Portsmouth, Hampshire
— Radcliffe Infirmary – Oxford
— Romsey Hospital - Romsey
— Royal Berkshire Hospital - Reading, Berkshire
— Royal Buckinghamshire Hospital - Aylesbury, Buckinghamshire
— Royal Hampshire County Hospital - Winchester
— Royal Hospital Haslar - Gosport, Hampshire
— Royal South Hampshire Hospital - Southampton
— Southampton General Hospital - Southampton
— Stoke Mandeville Hospital - Aylesbury, Buckinghamshire
— St Christopher's Hospital - Fareham, Hampshire

- St James' Hospital - Portsmouth, Hampshire
- St Mary's Hospital - Isle of Wight
- St Mary's Hospital - Portsmouth, Hampshire
- Tatchbury Mount Hospital - Totton
- Western Hospital - Southampton
- Wexham Park Hospital - Wexham, Slough, Berkshire
- Ashford Hospital - Ashford, Surrey
- St Peter's Hospital - Chertsey, Surrey

South West

- Bristol Royal Infirmary - Bristol
- Cheltenham General Hospital - Cheltenham, Gloucestershire
- Derriford Hospital - Plymouth
- Frenchay Hospital - Bristol
- Gloucester Royal Hospital - Gloucester
- Great Western Hospital - Swindon
- North Devon District Hospital - Barnstaple, Devon
- Paulton Memorial Hospital - Paulton, Somerset
- Royal Cornwall Hospital - Truro
- Royal Devon and Exeter Hospital - Exeter
- Royal National Hospital for Rheumatic Diseases - Bath
- Royal United Hospital - Bath, Somerset
- Southmead Hospital - Bristol
- Stoke Military Hospital - Plymouth (closed in 1945)
- The Old Manor Hospital - Salisbury
- Torbay District Hospital - Torquay
- Weston General Hospital - Weston-super-Mare, North Somerset

West Midlands

- Birmingham Children's Hospital - Birmingham
- City Hospital, Birmingham - Birmingham

- — Good Hope Hospital - Sutton Coldfield
- — Heartlands Hospital - Birmingham
- — New Cross Hospital - Wolverhampton
- — Princess Royal Hospital - Telford
- — Queen Elizabeth Hospital - Birmingham
- — Robert Jones and Agnes Hunt Orthopaedic Hospital - Oswestry
- — Royal Shrewsbury Hospital - Shrewsbury
- — Selly Oak Hospital - Birmingham
- — Stafford General Hospital
- — University Hospital of North Staffordshire - Stoke-on-Trent
- — University Hospital Coventry - Coventry (Opened 2006 as a replacement for Walsgrave Hospital & Coventry and Warwichshire Hospital)
- — Yorkshire and the Humber
- — North and East Yorkshire and Northern Lincolnshire Strategic Health Authority
- — Alfred Bean Hospital - Driffield, East Riding of Yorkshire
- — Bridlington and District Hospital - Bridlington, East Riding of Yorkshire
- — Castle Hill Hospital - Cottingham, East Riding of Yorkshire
- — Diana Princess of Wales Hospital - Grimsby, North East Lincolnshire
- — Goole and District Hospital - Goole, East Riding of Yorkshire
- — Harrogate District Hospital - Harrogate, North Yorkshire
- — Hull and East Riding Hospital - Anlaby, Hull, East Riding of Yorkshire

— Hull Nuffield Hospital - Cottingham, East Riding of Yorkshire
— Hull Royal Infirmary - Hull, East Riding of Yorkshire
— Malton Community Hospital - Malton, North Yorkshire
— The Retreat - York, North Yorkshire
— Ripon and District Community Hospital - Ripon, North Yorkshire
— St Hugh's Hospital - Grimsby, North East Lincolnshire
— Scarborough General Hospital - Scarborough, North Yorkshire
— Whitby Community Hospital - Whitby, North Yorkshire
— York Hospital - York, North Yorkshire
— South Yorkshire Strategic Health Authority
— Barnsley Hospital - Barnsley
— Charles Clifford Dental Hospital - Sheffield
— Doncaster Gate Hospital - Rotherham
— Doncaster Royal Infirmary - Doncaster
— Montagu Hospital - Mexborough
— Northern General Hospital - Sheffield
— Park Hill Hospital - Doncaster
— Rotherham District General Hospital - Rotherham
— Royal Hallamshire Hospital - Sheffield
— Sheffield Children's Hospital - Sheffield
— West Yorkshire Strategic Health Authority
— Airedale General Hospital - Keighley
— Bradford Royal Infirmary - Bradford
— Calderdale Royal Hospital - Halifax
— Castleford, Normanton and District Hospital - Castleford
— Chapel Allerton Hospital - Leeds
— Clayton Hospital - Wakefield
— Dewsbury and District Hospital - Dewsbury
— Leeds Dental Hospital - Leeds

— Leeds General Infirmary - Leeds
— Lynfield Mount Hospital - Bradford
— Huddersfield Royal Infirmary - Huddersfield
— Methley Park Hospital - Methley
— Nuffield Hospital Leeds - Leeds
— Pinderfields General Hospital - Wakefield
— Pontefract General Infirmary - Pontefract
— St James's University Hospital - Leeds
— St Luke's Hospital, Bradford - Bradford
— St Luke's Hospital, Huddersfield - Huddersfield
— Seacroft Hospital - Leeds
— Wharfedale Hospital – Otley

LIST OF HOSPITALS IN FRANCE

— Amiens University Hospital- Amiens
— Angers University Hospital- Angers
— Centre hospitalier universitaire de Caen- Caen
— Hôpital d'instruction des armées Percy- Clamart
— Grenoble University Hospital- Grenoble
— Limoges University Hospital- Limoges
— Claude Bernard University Hospital- Lyon
— Henri Poincaré University Hospital- Nancy
— Nantes University Hospital- Nantes
— Broussais University Hospital- Paris
— Hospital Europeen Georges Pompidou- Paris
— Institution Nationale des Invalides - Paris
— Necker University Hospital- Paris
— Pitié-Salpêtrière Hospital - Paris
— Saint-Antoine University Hospital- Paris
— Val-de-Grâce military hospital- Paris
— Reims University Hospital- Reims
— Rennes University Hospital- Rennes

— Rouen University Hospital- Rouen
— Tourcoing Hospital- Tourcoing

LIST OF HOSPITALS IN GERMANY

— Klinikum Aachen
— Charité Universitätsmedizin Berlin
— Berufsgenossenschaftliche Kliniken Bergmannsheil Bochum
— Rheinische_Friedrich-Wilhelms-University Hospital Bonn
— University Hospital Essen
— University Hospital Frankfurt a.M.
— University Hospital Freiburg
— University Hospital Gießen and Marburg
— University Hospital Halle
— University Hospital Hamburg-Eppendorf
— Medical School Hannover
— University Hospital Heidelberg
— University Hospital Heidelberg
— University Hospital of the Saarland, Homburg (Saar)
— University Hospital Köln
— University Hospital Leipzig
— University Hospital Magdeburg
— University Hospital Mainz
— University Hospital Marburg
— University Hospital Großhadern
— University Hospital Rechts der Isar
— University Hospital Münster
— University Hospital Schleswig-Holstein (Lübeck and Kiel)
— Eberhard-Karls-University Hospital Tübingen
— University Hospital Ulm
— University Hospital Würzburg

LIST OF HOSPITALS IN HONG KONG

Hospitals and Institutions Managed by the Hospital Authority

Hong Kong West Cluster

- Queen Mary Hospital
- Tsan Yuk Hospital
- Tung Wah Hospital
- Tung Wah Group of Hospitals - Fung Yiu King Hospital
- The Duchess of Kent Children's Hospital at Sandy Bay
- MacLehose Medical Rehabilitation Centre
- Grantham Hospital
- Nam Long Hospital

Hong Kong East Cluster

- Pamela Youde Nethersole Eastern Hospital
- Tang Shiu Kin Hospital
- Ruttonjee Hospital
- Tung Wah Eastern Hospital
- St. John Hospital
- Cheshire Home, Chung Hom Kok
- Wong Chuk Hang Hospital

Kowloon Central Cluster

- Queen Elizabeth Hospital
- Kowloon Hospital
- Hong Kong Buddhist Hospital
- HK Red Cross Blood Transfusion Service
- Hong Kong Eye Hospital
- Rehabaid Centre

Kowloon West Cluster

- Kwong Wah Hospital
- TWGHs Wong Tai Sin Hospital

— Our Lady of Maryknoll Hospital
— Caritas Medical Centre
— Kwai Chung Hospital
— Princess Margaret Hospital
— Yan Chai Hospital

Kowloon East Cluster

— United Christian Hospital
— Haven of Hope Hospital
— Tseung Kwan O Hospital

New Territories East Cluster

— Prince of Wales Hospital
— Shatin Hospital
— Cheshire Home, Shatin
— Bradbury Hospice
— Alice Ho Miu Ling Nethersole Hospital
— Tai Po Hospital
— North District Hospital

New Territories West Cluster

— Tuen Mun Hospital
— Pok Oi Hospital
— Castle Peak Hospital
— Siu Lam Hospital

Private Hospitals

— Baptist Hospital
— Evangel Hospital
— Hong Kong Adventist Hospital
— Hong Kong Central Hospital
— Hong Kong Sanatorium and Hospital
— Matilda International Hospital
— Precious Blood Hospital

— St. Paul's Hospital
— St. Teresa's Hospital (commonly known to locals as the "French Hospital")
— Tsuen Wan Adventist Hospital
— Union Hospital

General Out-Patient Clinics

Hong Kong Island

— Aberdeen Jockey Club Clinic
— Sai Ying Pun Jockey Club General Outpatient Clinic
— Shau Kei Wan Jockey Club Clinic
— Violet Peel Health Centre

Kowloon Region

— Central Kowloon Health Centre
— Cheung Sha Wan Jockey Club General Out-patient Clinic
— Kwun Tong Jockey Club Health Centre
— Lady Trench General Out-patient Clinic
— Li Po Chun General Out-patient Clinic
— Robert Black General Out-patient Clinic
— Yau Ma Tei Jockey Club Clinic

New Territories Region

— Lek Yuen Health Centre
— Ma On Shan Health Centre
— Shek Wu Hui Jockey Club Clinic
— Tseung Kwan O Po Ning Rd, Health Centre
— Tung Chung General Out-patient Clinic
— Tsing Yi Cheung Hong General Outpatient Clinic
— Tuen Mun Clinic
— Yuen Long Jockey Club Health Centre
— Tin Shui Wai Health Centre

LIST OF HOSPITALS IN IRAN

Tehran Province

- 17 Shahrivar
- 22nd of Bahman
- 502 Artesh
- 503 Artesh
- 504 Artesh
- 505 Artesh
- 506 Artesh
- Akhtar Hospital
- Alghadir
- Ali Asghar
- Alvand
- Amin Sadeghiyeh (Zayeshgah)
- Amir Aalam
- Amir Almoaamenin
- AmirAlmomenin
- Andarzgo
- Arad Hospital
- Atieh Hospital
- Ayatollah Kashani
- Ayatollah Khansari
- Ayatollah Taleghani
- Azadi Psychiatric Hospital
- Babak (Zayeshgah)
- Baghiyatolah Aazam
- Baharlo
- Baher Hospital
- Bahrami
- Bank Meli Iran
- Boali Hospital
- Bozorgmehr

— Chehrazy Hospital
— Cheshm Pezeshkieh Payambaran
— Dadgostari
— Day Hospital
— Dr Maseh Daneshvari
— Dr Moairi
— Dr. Razmi
— Dr Sepir
— Eghbal (Zayeshgah)
— Emam Hosein
— Esmaili (Ravani)
— Eyvaz Zadeh
— Fajr Hospital
— Farabi (Cheshm)
— Farabi Jadid
— Firozabadi
— Gamaran (heart)
— Ghiyasi
— Hashemi Nejad
— Hazrate Fatemeh Zahra
— Hazrate Mohammad
— Hoseyniyeh Ershad
— Imam Khomeini Hospital Center
— Imam Hossein
— Iran Hospital
— Iranmehr
— Jam
— Javahery
— Jorjani Hospital
— Khanevadeh (Artesh)
— Khatam Hospital
— Khatamolanbia

— Kian Hospital (Kyan General Hospital)
— Laleh Hospital
— Loghman Hakim (Masmomeat)
— Lolagar Hospital
— Madaen
— Madar Hospital
— Madaran Hospital
— Mahdieh
— Mardom
— Marghad Shahr
— MarvastiHospital
— Mehrad Hospital
— Meymanat
— Milad Hospital
— Modares (heart)
— Mofarah Hospital
— Mofid Hospital
— Moghoufeh Nouh
— Najmiyeh
— Nasr
— Nirooye Entezami No.2
— Nirooye Entezami No.1
— Nirooye daryayi
— Nirooye Havaei
— No.5 Shahid Fayaz Bakhsh
— Noor Afshar
— Noor Saadat
— Noor Vision Correction Center
— Omid Hospital
— Park Killinik
— Parsian Hospital
— Pasargad
— Payambaran

— Rajayi
— Razi (Razani)
— Razi Hospital
— Resalat Hospital
— Rezaei (Asab and Ravan)
— Roen Tan Arash
— Roozbeh Hospital
— Sevom Shaban
— Seyedolshohada
— Shafa Yahyaian
— Shahid Andarzgou
— Shahid Ashrafi esfahani
— Shahid Dr Chamran
— Shahid Dr Lavasani
— Shahid Fahmideh
— Shahid Labafi Nejad
— Shahid Mottahari (sookhtegi)
— Shahid Rajayi
— Shahid Shariat Razavi
— Shahriar Hospital
— Shariati
— Sherkat Naft
— Shohaday Yaft Abad
— Shohadaye Hafte Tir
— Shohadaye Larzan
— Shohadaye Tajrish
— Sina Hospital
— Takhti (Kodakan)
— Tavanbakhshi-e Malolin-e Zehni (vezarat Kar and Omur Ejtemai)
— Tehran Pars
— Torfeh Hospital
— Tus Hospital

- Valiasr Hospital
- Vasei Hospital
- Yaser Hospital
- Ziaeian

LIST OF HOSPITALS IN ITALY

- San Raffaele Hospital - Milan
- Azienda Ospedaliera Papardo - Messina
- Bologna Public Health Departments - Bologna
- Burlo Garofolo Pediatric Institute - Trieste
- Careggi Hospital of University of Florence - Florence
- Cattinara Hospital - Trieste
- Mauro Leonardis - Rome
- Orthopedic Institute Gaetano Pini - Milan
- S.Camillo Zonal Hospital - Treviso
- San Giovanni di Dio Hospital - Florence
- Azienda Sanitaria di Modena - Modena
- United States Naval Station Hospital - Naples
- San Camillo Forlanini - Rome
- Le Molinette – Turin

LIST OF HOSPITALS IN KENYA

This is a list of hospitals in Kenya.

This list is incomplete; you can help by expanding it.

- Diani Beach Hospital - Mombasa
- Mombasa Hospital- Mombasa
- Ojele Memorial Hospital- Suna
- Kenyatta National Hospital Nairobi
- Nairobi Hospital Nairobi
- Aga Khan Memorial Hospital
- Provincial General Hospital

— Kijabe Hospital
— The Mater hospital,Nairobi,Kenya
— Kisii District Hospital
— Moi Teaching and Refferal Hospital, Eldoret

LIST OF HOSPITALS IN NIGERIA

From Wikipedia, the free encyclopedia

Akwa Ibom State

— St.Lukes Hospital,Ituk Mbang,Uruan
— University of Uyo Teaching Hospital
— State Hospital Anua
— Emmanuel Hospital ,Eket
— General Hospital ,Oron
— General Hospital Etinan

Anambra State

— Nnamdi Azikiwe University Teaching Hospital, Nnewi, Anambra
— St. Charles Borromeo Hospital, Onitsha

Benue State

— Madonna Hospital, Makurdi - http://madonnahospital.com/
— St Luke's Hospital, Gboko

Cross River State

— General Hospital, Calabar, Cross River
— Holy Family Hospital, Ikom, Cross River

Edo State

— Central Hospital, Benin, Edo
— University of Benin Teaching Hospital, Ugbowo, Benin, Edo State.

- Benoni Hospital Nigeria Ltd, Boundary Road, Benin, Edo State
- Neuro-Psychiatric Hospital, Uselu, Benin City

Cross River State

- University of Calabar Teaching Hospital, Moore Road, Calabar, CRS
- University of Calabar Teaching Hospital, Etar Agbor Road, Calabar, CRS

Enugu State

- National Orthopedic Hospital, Enugu
- Niger Foundation Hospital, Enugu
- University of Nigeria Teaching Hospital, Enugu

Federal Capital Territory

- National Hospital, Abuja
- Zankli Medical Centre, Abuja
- Hugo Medical Center, Abuja
- Wuse General Hospital, Abuja
- St. Mary's Catholic Hospital, Gwagwalada, Abuja
- [http://www.abujaclinics.com Abuja Clinic
- Nisa premier Hospital, Jabi,Abuja

Kano State

- Infectious Disease Hospital, Kano
- Murtala Mohammed Specialist Hospital, Kano

Kwara State

- University of Ilorin Teaching Hospital, Ilorin
- Omolola Hopsital, Ilorin
- OlaOlu Hospital, Ilorin
- Sobi Specialist Hospital, Sobi, Ilorin
- Olanrewaju hospital, Ilorin
- Hassanat Memorial Hospital

— Surulere Medical Center
— Anchor Clinic
— Eyitayo Clinic
— Delnic Clinic

Lagos

— A And A Medical Diagnostic Centre, Ishaga Road, Surulere,
— AB Specialist Clinic, Tinubu Square, Lagos Island
— Active Health Managers Limited, Dolphin Estate, Ikoyi, Lagos
— Agage General Hospital
— Alalade Memorial Hospital, Ijesatedo, Lagos
— All Souls Clinics Limited, Ojo Road, Mile 2, Ajegunle, Apapa, Lagos
— Apapa general Hospital
— Ayo-Ade Oshin Memorial Hospital and Maternity Home, Hawley Street, Lagos
— Badagari General Hospital
— BAF Eye Centre Ltd, Oba Adetona Street, Off Sura Mogaji Street, Ilupeju, Lagos
— Barnes Diagnostic And Heart Centre, Ajose Adeogun Street,
— Bimax Hospital and Maternity Home, Surulere Street,, Dopemu-Agege, Lagos
— Bob Specialist Hospital Limited, Olugbende Street, Off Idimu Street,
— Brume Sankey Surgical Nig. Ltd, Stephen Osibote Close, Okoto Layout, Isolo, Lagos
— Chromeu Medical Centre, Olufemi Samson Street, Okomalam, Lagos
— Christ Medical Centre, Randle Road, Apapa, Lagos
— Clear view Optics Ltd, Alhaji Ribadu Road, South-West Ikoyi, Lagos

- — Crest Consultant Clinic, Keffi Street, South-West Ikoyi, Lagos
- — Dolfac Medical Centre, Ibukun-Olu Street, Akoka, Lagos
- — Dortem Specialist Hospital, Babs Animashhun Road, Surulere, Lagos
- — Duro Soleye Hospitals, Allen Avenue, Ikeja, Lagos
- — Ebutameta Health Center
- — Ekemode Memorial Hospital and Women's Infi, Bode Thomas Street, Surulere, Lagos
- — Eko Hospital, Mobolaji Bank Anthony Way, Ikeja, Lagos
- — First Consultancy Medical Centre, Obalende, Lagos
- — First Foundation Medical Company Ltd, Opebi Road, Ikeja, Lagos
- — Gbolayemi Clinic, Ladipo Oluwole Street, Apapa, Lagos
- — General Medical Care, Ologun Agbaje Street, Victoria Island, Lagos
- — Global Medical Centre Services, Ologun Agbaje Street, Victoria Island, Lagos
- — Gloryland Clinc, Odo Olowu Street, Via Apapa-Oshodi Express Way, Lagos
- — Gold Cross Hospital, Keffi Street, South-West Ikoyi, Lagos
- — Havana Specialist Hospital Ltd, Akerele Street (Teslim Fatusi Street), Surulere, Lagos
- — Hugo Medical Center, Lagos
- — Iganmu Industrial Clinic, Eric Moore Close, Iganmu, Surulere, Lagos
- — Ikeja General Hospital
- — Isolo General hospital
- — Jalupon Estate Hospital, Bode Thomas Street, Surulere, Lagos

— Joas Medical Diagnostix, Joas House, Ikotun, Lagos
— Kings Foundation Clinic Ltd, Olutoye Crescent, Off Adeniyi Jones Avenue, Lagos
— Landay Satellite Clinic, Apapa Amusement Park, Apapa, Lagos
— Lafia Group Hospital, Wharf Road (Development House), Apapa, Lagos
— Lagoon Hospital, Marine Road, Apapa
— Lagoon Hospital, Balogun Street, Ikeja, Lagos
— Lagos General Hospital
— Lagos Mainland Hospital, Lagos
— Lagos University Teaching Hospital
— Leo Specialist Hospital, Balogun Street, Lagos
— Lifeline Children Hospital, Ogunlana Drive, Surulere, Lagos
— Little Way Clinic, Moshalasi Street, Obalende, Lagos
— Macey Medical Centre, Capricorn Block Ground Floor, Eleganza Plaza, Apapa, Lagos
— Madikem Clinic, Sobo Arobiodu Street, GRA, Ikeja, Lagos
— Mainland Hospital, Marina, Lagos
— Marantha Hospital, St. Finbarr's College Road, Akoka, Yaba, Lagos
— Martins Hospital, Lagos-Abeokuta Express Road, Anya Bus-Stop, Alagbado, Lagos
— Massey Street Children's Hospital, Lagos
— May Hospitals & Specialist Clinics Ltd, Lagos
— Maydelen Hospital, Araotic Street, Yaba, Lagos
— Medical Clinics Maternity Home, Abibu Oki Street, Lagos
— Military Hospital Ikoyi
— Motayo Hospital Services Ltd, Owodunni Street, Off Toyin Street, Ikeja, Lagos

- Mother & Child Hospitals, Adeniyi Jones, Ikeja, Lagos
- Mount Sanai Hospital Ltd, Borno Way, Ebute-Metta, Lagos
- Mt. Zion Specialist Clinic, Adeolu Street, Surulere, Lagos
- National Orthopaedic Hospital,Igbobi,Lagos
- National Orthopaedic Hospital
- Neuro-Psychiatric Hospital, Yaba, Lagos
- O & S Hospitals, Lagos
- Okiki Clinic and Maternity Hospital, Lagos, Lagos State
- Oluwatoyin Clinic,Ojota,Lagos
- Oshodi Tapa Memorial Hospital, Imam Dauda Street, Off Eric More, Surulere, Lagos
- Parklande Specialist Hospital, Lagos
- Pipe Street Medical Centre, Pike Street, Lagos
- Plato Hospital, Shogunle, Lagos
- Premier Hospital, Ogalode Close, Victoria Island, Lagos
- Providence Hospital, Itire Road, Surulere, Lagos
- R-Jolad Hospital
- Roland Hospital, Joseph Street, Lagos
- Rotfol Medical Centre, Atunrase Street, Off Ishaga Road, Surulere, Lagos
- Saraki-Ikomi Group Clinics, Kofo Abayomi Avenue, Apapa, Lagos
- Shigun Hospital,Ilupeju,Lagos
- Solid Rock Hospital, Ojodu, Lagos
- St. Charles Hospitals Limited, Ayilara Street, Surulere, Lagos
- St. Francis Hospital, Keffi Street, South-West Ikoyi, Lagos
- St. George Hospital Ltd., Makinde Road, Surulere, Lagos

— St. Georges Medical Centre, 6,Rasheed Alaba William St.Off Admirality, Lekki Phase I, Lagos
— St. Ives Hospitals, Opebi, Ikeja, Lagos
— St. Louise Medical Centre, Prince Court, Victoria Island, Lagos
— St. Louise Clinic, Abibu Oki Street, Lagos
— St. Nicolas Hospital, Campbell Street, Lagos Island, Lagos
— St. Thelma's Hospital & Maternity Home, Anuoluwapo Street, Bariga, Lagos
— Surulere General Hospital
— Syl Memorial Hospital Akeem Akonju St. Ikeja
— Teboree Clinic, Tokunbo Street, Lagos
— Teju Industries Clinc Ltd, Creek Road, Apapa, Lagos
— The Clinic, Apena Street, Surulere, Lagos
— Timu Hospital Group, Mushin Road, Isolo, Lagos
— Tolu Hospital, Old Abeokuta Road, Apapa, Lagos
— University Teaching Hospital, Lagos
— Vincent Maternity, Ikeja, Lagos
— White Chapel Hospital Ltd, Adebisi Awosoga Street, Dopemu-Agege, Lagos
— White Chapel Hospital Ltd, Obafemi Awolowo Way, Ikeja, Lagos
— Yaba Medical Centre, Agard Street, Yaba, Lagos
— Zenith Clinic, Kakawa Street, Lagos
— St. Georges Medical Centre, 6,Rasheed Alaba William St.Off Admirality, Lekki Phase I, Lagos

Osun State

— Obafemi Awolowo University Teaching Hospital Complex
— Seventh Day Adventist Hospital

Owo

— Federal Medical Centre

Plateau State

— Jos University Teaching Hospital, Jos
— Adoose Specialist Hospital, Jos
— ECWA Evangel Hospital, Jos

LIST OF HOSPITALS IN SOUTH AFRICA

This is a list of hospitals in South Africa.

Eastern Cape

East London

— East London Private Hospital
— St Dominic's Hospital
— St James Hospital

Port Elizabeth

— Greenacres Hospital
— Hunterscraig Private Hospital
— Mercantile Hospital
— Oasim Private Hospital
— St George's Hospital
— Westways Private Hospital

Umtata

— St Mary's Private Hospital
— Umtata General Hospital

Other

— Cecilia Makiwane
— Grey Monument Private Clinic (King William's Town)
— Cuyler Hospital (Uitenhage)

Free State

Bloemfontein

— Bloemfontein Medi-Clinic
— Pelonomi Hospital
— Rosepark Hospital
— Universitas Hospital

Other

— Ernest Oppenheimer Hospital (Welkom)
— Hoogland Medi-Clinic (Bethlehem)
— Welkom Medi-Clinic (Welkom)
— Kroon Hospital (Kroonstad)

Gauteng

Johannesburg

— Bedford Gardens Clinic
— Chris Hani Baragwanath Hospital
— Coronation Hospital
— Garden City Hospital
— Helen Joseph Hospital
— Johannesburg General Hospital
— Leratong Hospital
— Linksfield Park Clinic
— Marymount Hospital
— Milpark Hospital
— Morningside Medi-Clinic
— Olivedale Clinic
— Sandton Medi-Clinic
— South Rand Hospital
— Sunninghill Hospital
— Tara Psychiatric Hospital
— Wilgeheuwel Hospital
— Wits University Donald Gordon Medical Centre

Pretoria

- Eugene Marais Hospital
- Faerie Glen Hospital
- Jacaranda Hospital
- Kalafong Hospital
- Kloof Medi-Clinic
- Little Company of Mary
- Louis Pasteur Hospital
- Medforum Medi-Clinic
- Medi-Clinic Gynaecological Hospital
- Medi-Clinic Heart Hospital
- Montana Hospital
- Muelmed Medi-Clinic
- Pretoria Academic Hospital
- Pretoria East Private Hospital
- Pretoria Eye Institute
- Pretoria Urology Hospital
- Unitas Hospital
- Weskoppies Psychiatric Hospital
- Wilgers Hospital
- Zuid-Afrikaans Hospital

Other

- Natalspruit Hospital
- Vereeniging Medi-Clinic (Vereeniging)
- Union Hospital (Alberton)
- Glynnwood Hospital (Benoni)
- Linmed Clinic (Benoni)
- Sunward Park Hospital (Boksburg)
- Lenmed Clinic (Lenasia)
- Carstenhof Clinic (Midrand)
- Robinson Hospital (Randfontein)

— Flora Clinic (Roodepoort)
— N17 Hospital (Springs)
— Springs Parkland Clinic (Springs)
— Midvaal Hospitaal (Vereeniging)
— Arwyp Clinic (Kempton Park)
— Bell Street Hospital (Krugersdorp)
— Krugersdorp Private Hospital (Krugersdorp)

KwaZulu-Natal

Durban

— Addington Hospital
— Chief Albert Luthuli Hospital
— Crompton Private Hospital
— Entabeni Hospital
— King Edward VIII Hospital
— Kingsway Private Hospital
— Mahatma Gandhi Memorial Hospital
— McCord Hospital
— Parklands Private Hospital
— Prince Mshiyeni Hospital
— St Augustine's Hospital
— Westville Private Hospital

Pietermaritzburg

— Grey's Hospital
— Edendale Hospital
— St Anne's Hospital
— Pietermaritzburg Medi-Clinic

Other

— Howick Private Hospital (Howick)
— Newcastle Private Hospital (Newcastle)

— Victoria Private Hospital (Tongaat)
— Margate Private Hospital (Margate)

Limpopo

Polokwane

— Limpopo Medi-Clinic
— Mankweng Hospital

Other

— Curamed Thabazimbi Hospital
— Tzaneen Private Hospital

Mpumalanga

Nelspruit

— Rob Ferreira Hospital
— Nelspruit Medi-Clinic

Other

— Barberton Medi-Clinic
— Ermelo Medi-Clinic
— Highveld Medi-Clinic
— Secunda Medi-Clinic
— Themba Hospital

Northern Cape

Kimberley

— Kimberley Medi-Clinic

Upington

— Upington Medi-Clinic

North West

Klerksdorp

— Anncron Clinic
— Wilmed Private Hospital

Other

— Brits Medi-Clinic - Brits
— Ferncrest Private Hospital -Tlhabane
— Legae Private Clinic - Mabopane
— Peglerae Private Hospital - Rustenburg
— Potchefstroom Medi-Clinic - Potchefstroom
— Victoria Private Hospital - Mafikeng

Western Cape

Cape Town

— Bellville Medical Centre
— Cape Town Medi-Clinic
— Christiaan Barnard Memorial Hospital
— Claremont Hospital
— Constantiaberg Medi-Clinic
— Groote Schuur Hospital
— False Bay Hospital
— Karl Bremmer Hospital
— Kingsbury Hospital
— Lentegeur Psychiatric Hospital
— Louis Leipoldt Medi-Clinic
— Milnerton Medi-Clinic
— Mitchells Plain Medical Centre
— N1 City Hospital
— Panorama Medi-Clinic
— Red Cross War Memorial Children's Hospital
— Somerset Hospital
— Valkenberg Psychiatric Hospital
— Vergelegen Medi-Clinic
— Victoria Hospital
— Vincent Pallotti Hospital

George

— Geneva Clinic
— George Medi-Clinic

Hermanus

— Hermanus Hospital
— Hermanus Medi-Clinic

Paarl

— Paarl Hospital
— Paarl Medi-Clinic

Stellenbosch

— Stellenbosch Hospital
— Stellenbosch Medi-Clinic

Worcester

— Eben Donges Hospital
— Worcester Medi-Clinic

Other

— Klein Karoo Medi-Clinic
— Knysna Private Hospital

LIST OF HOSPITALS IN SPAIN

— Hospital Universitario La Paz Link - Madrid
— Clinica Moncloa - Madrid
— Clinica Universitaria de Navarra - Pamplona
— Corporación Parc Taulí - Sabadell
— Fundación Hospital Verín - Verín
— Fundacion Hospital Alcorcón - Madrid
— Hospital de Albacete - Albacete
— Hospital de Basurto - Bilbao
— Hospital de Cabueñes - Gijon
— Hospital de Cruces - Barakaldo

— Hospital Juan Canalejo - A Coruña
— Hospital de Móstoles - Móstoles, Madrid
— Hospital Universitari Son Dureta - Palma de Mallorca

LIST OF HOSPITALS IN THAILAND

Bangkok

— Bangkok Hospital (Bangkok General Hospital), 2 Soi Soonvijai 7, New Petchaburi Road,
— Bangkok Christian Hospital, 124 Silom Road, Bang Rak
— Bangkok Mission Hospital, 430 Pitsanulok Road, Dusit
— Bhumibol Adulyadej Hospital, 171 Paholyothin Road, Don Mueang
— BNH Hospital (Bangkok Nursing Home Hospital), 9/ 1 Convent Road,
— Bumrungrad Hospital - international medical tourism center located at 33 Sukhumvit Road Soi 3, Watthana
— Camillian Hospital, 423 Soi Thong Lo, Watthana
— Chao Phaya Hospital, Pinklao Road, Thon Buri
— King Chulalongkorn Memorial Hospital, 1873 Rama IV Road
— Kasemrad Prachachuen Hospital, 950 Prachachuen Road, Bang Sue
— Kluaynamthai General Hospital
— Monkuwattana Hospital, near International School Bangkok, 34/40 Chaengwattana Road, Lak Si
— Paolo Memorial Hospital, 670/1 Paholyothin Road
— Phayathai 1 Hospital, 364 Sri Ayuthaya Road
— Phayathai 2 Hospital, 943 Petchkasem Road, Pakklong
— Phayathai 3 Hospital, 207/26 Petchkasem Road, Thon Buri
— Police General Hospital, 492/1 Rama I Road, Pathum Wan

— Pramongkutklao Hospital, 315 Rajavithi Road, Phaya Thai
— Praram 9 Hospital, Rama IX Road
— Promitr Hospital, 12 Sukhumvit Road Soi 39, Watthana
— Ramathibodi University Hospital, 270 Rama VI Road
— Siriraj Hospital, 2 Prannok Road, Thon Buri
— St. Louis Hospital- Yannawa
— Samitivej Hospital, 133 Sukhumvit Road Soi 49 Watthana
— Theptarin Hospital, 3850 Rama IV Road
— Thonburi Hospital
— Vichaiyut Hospital, 114/4 Setsiri Road, Phaya Thai

Chiang Mai

— McCormick Hospital
— Chiangmai Ram Hospital
— Chiang Mai Ram 2 Hospital
— Chang Phuak Hospital
— Chiang Mai Central Memorial Hospital
— Chiang Mai Dental Hospital
— Chiang Mai Neurological Hosptial
— Chinda Hospital
— Dararasmi Hospital
— Dr. Wong Hospital
— Klai Mor Hospital
— Lanna Hospital
— Maharaj Hospital
— McKene Rehabilitation Center
— Nakornping Hospital
— Rajavej Chiang Mai Hospital
— Ruam Padh Hospital
— St.Peter Eye Hospital
— Vector Borne Disease Control 2

Khon Kaen

— Khon Kaen Ram

— Sri Nagarind Hospital - Khon Kaen

Pattaya

— Bangkok Pattaya Hospital, Sukhumvit Road (*immediately north-west of the North Pattaya Road traffic lights* - 210 beds) website / website / inquiry@bph.co.th tel. 038-259999 / emergencies: 038-259911

— Banglamung Hospital, Sawang Fah Road, Naklua - tel. 038-429244 /5 (the least foreigner-orientated of Pattaya's major hospitals)

— Pattaya International Hospital, Soi 4 (*between Pattaya Beach Road and Second Road, North Pattaya*) website / picpih@loxinfo.co.th tel. 038-428374 /5

— Pattaya Memorial Hospital, Central Pattaya Road - tel. 038-429422 /4 (has the most central location, but does not have as good a reputation as Bangkok Pattaya Hospital or Pattaya International Hospital)

Phuket

— Phuket International Hospital- website / tel. +66 76 249400

— Bangkok Phuket Hospital

— Mission Hospital

— Patong Hospital

Trang

— Trang Ruampat Hospital

5

Select List of Diseases

A

— Aagenaes syndrome
— Aarskog Ose Pande syndrome
— Aarskog syndrome
— Aase Smith syndrome
— Aase syndrome
— ABCD syndrome
— Abdallat Davis Farrage syndrome
— Abdominal aortic aneurysm
— Abdominal cystic lymphangioma
— Abdominal defects
— Abdominal musculature absent microphthalmia joint laxity
— Abdominal neoplasms
— Aberrant subclavian artery
— Ablepharon macrostomia syndrome
— Abnormal systemic venous return
— Abruzzo Erickson syndrome
— Absence of Gluteal muscle
— Absence of tibia with polydactyly
— Absent corpus callosum cataract immunodeficiency
— Absent T lymphocytes
— Acalvaria
— Acanthocheilonemiasis
— Acanthocytosis chorea
— Acanthocytosis
— Acanthosis nigricans
— Acatalasemia
— Accessory deep peroneal nerve

— Accessory Navicular bone
— Accessory pancreas
— Achalasia alacrimia syndrome
— Achalasia microcephaly
— Achalasia, familial esophageal
— Achalasia
— Achalasia-Addisonianism-Alacrimia syndrome
— Achard syndrome
— Achard-Thiers syndrome
— Acheiropodia
— Achondrogenesis Kozlowski type
— Achondrogenesis
— Achondroplasia Swiss type agammaglobulinemia
— Achondroplasia
— Achondroplastic dwarfism
— Achromatopsia incomplete, X-linked
— Achromatopsia
— Acid maltase deficiency
— Acidemia, isovaleric
— Acidemia, propionic
— Acitretine antenatal infection
— Ackerman syndrome
— Acne
— Acoustic neuroma
— Acoustic schwannomas
— Acquired agranulocytosis
— Acquired hypoprothrombinemia
— Acquired Immune Deficiency Syndrome
— Acquired ichthyosis
— Acquired prothrombin deficiency
— Acquired syphilis
— Acral dysostosis dyserythropoiesis
— Acral renal mandibular syndrome
— Acro coxo mesomelic dysplasia
— Acro fronto facio nasal dysostosis
— Acrocallosal syndrome, Schinzel type
— Acrocephalopolydactyly
— Acrocephalosyndactyly Jackson Weiss type
— Acrocephaly pulmonary stenosis mental retardation
— Acrodermatitis enteropathica

— Acrodermatitis
— Acrodysostosis
— Acrodysplasia scoliosis
— Acrofacial dysostosis ambiguous genitalia
— Acrofacial dysostosis atypical postaxial
— Acrofacial dysostosis Catania form
— Acrofacial dysostosis Preis type
— Acrofacial dysostosis Rodriguez type
— Acrofacial dysostosis Weyers type
— Acrofacial dysostosis, Nager type
— Acrofacial dysostosis, Palagonia type
— Acrokeratoelastoidosis of Costa
— Acromegaloid changes cutis verticis gyrata corneal
— Acromegaloid facial appearance syndrome
— Acromegaloid hypertrichosis syndrome
— Acromegaly
— Acromesomelic dysplasia Brahimi Bacha type
— Acromesomelic dysplasia Campailla Martinelli type
— Acromesomelic dysplasia Hunter Thompson type
— Acromesomelic dysplasia, Maroteaux type
— Acromesomelic dysplasia
— Acromicric dysplasia
— Acroosteolysis dominant type
— Acroosteolysis neurogenic
— Acroosteolysis osteoporosis skull and mandible changes
— Acropectoral syndrome
— Acropectorenal field defect
— Acropectorovertebral dysplasia
— Acrophobia
— Acropigmentation of Dohi
— Acrorenal syndrome recessive
— Acrorenoocular syndrome
— Acrospiroma
— ACTH deficiency
— ACTH resistance
— Atelectasis
— Actinic keratosis
— Actinomycetales infection
— Actinomycosis
— Activated protein C resistance

— Acutane embryopathy
— Acute articular rheumatism
— Acute erythroblastic leukemia
— Acute febrile neutrophilic dermatosis
— Acute gouty arthritis
— Acute idiopathic polyneuritis
— Acute intermittent porphyria
— Acute lymphoblastic leukemia congenital sporadic aniridia
— Acute lymphoblastic leukemia
— Acute lymphocytic leukemia
— Acute megakaryoblastic leukemia
— Acute monoblastic leukemia
— Acute monocytic leukemia
— Acute mountain sickness
— Acute myeloblastic leukemia
— Acute myeloblastic leukemia with maturation
— Acute myeloblastic leukemia without maturation
— Acute myelocytic leukemia
— Acute myelogenous leukemia
— Acute myeloid leukemia (generic term)
— Acute myeloid leukemia, secondary
— Acute myelomonocytic leukemia
— Acute necrotizing ulcerative gingivitis
— Acute non lymphoblastic leukemia (generic term)
— Acute pancreatitis
— Acute posterior multifocal placoid pigment epitheliopathy
— Acute promyelocytic leukemia
— Acute renal failure
— Acute respiratory distress syndrome
— Acute tubular necrosis
— Acyl-CoA dehydrogenase, medium chain, deficiency of
— Acyl-CoA dehydrogenase, short chain, deficiency of
— Acyl-CoA dehydrogenase, very long chain, deficiency of
— Acyl-CoA oxidase deficiency
— Adactylia unilateral dominant
— Adam complex familial
— Adams Nance syndrome
— Adams-Oliver syndrome
— Addison's disease
— Adducted thumb club foot syndrome

— Adducted thumb syndrome recessive form
— Adducted thumbs Dundar type
— Adenine phosphoribosyltransferase deficiency
— Adenocarcinoid tumor
— Adenocarcinoma of lung
— Adenoid cystic carcinoma
— Adenoma of the adrenal gland
— Adenoma
— Adenomelablastoma
— Adenomyosis
— Adenosine deaminase deficiency
— Adenosine monophosphate deaminase deficiency
— Adenosine triphosphatase deficiency, anemia due to
— Adenylosuccinate lyase deficiency
— Adie syndrome
— Adiposis dolorosa aka Dercum's disease
— Adolescent benign focal crisis
— Adrenal adenoma, familial
— Adrenal cancer
— Adrenal disorder
— Adrenal gland hyperfunction
— Adrenal gland hypofunction
— Adrenal hyperplasia, congenital
— Adrenal hyperplasia
— Adrenal hypertension
— Adrenal hypoplasia congenital, X-linked
— Adrenal hypoplasia
— Adrenal incidentaloma
— Adrenal insufficiency
— Adrenal macropolyadenomatosis
— Adrenal medulla neoplasm
— Adrenocortical carcinoma
— Adrenogenital syndrome
— Adrenoleukodystrophy, autosomal, neonatal form
— Adrenoleukodystrophy, X-linked
— Adrenoleukodystrophy
— Adrenomyodystrophy
— Adult onset Still's disease
— Adult spinal muscular atrophy
— Adult syndrome

— Afibrinogenemia
— Aganglionosis, total intestinal
— Aging
— Aggressive fibromatosis
— Agnathia holoprosencephaly situs inversus
— Agnosia, primary visual
— Agoraphobia
— Agyria pachygyria polymicrogyria
— AIDS Dementia Complex
— AIDS dysmorphic syndrome
— Ainhum
— Akaba Hayasaka syndrome
— Albinism
— Albinoidism
— Albrecht Schneider Belmont syndrome
— Albright like syndrome
— Albright Turner Morgani syndrome
— Albright's hereditary osteodystrophy
— Albright's syndrome
— Alcaptonuria
— Alcohol antenatal infection
— Alcohol fetopathy
— Alcoholic hepatitis
— Alcoholic liver cirrhosis
— Aldolase A deficiency
— Aldred syndrome
— Aleukemic leukemia cutis
— Alexander disease
— Alien hand syndrome
— Alkaptonuria
— Allain Babin Demarquez syndrome
— Allan Herndon syndrome
— Allanson Pantzar McLeod syndrome
— Allergic angiitis
— Allergic autoimmune thyroiditis
— Allergic bronchopulmonary aspergillosis
— Allergic encephalomyelitis
— Aloi Tomasini Isaia syndrome
— Alopecia anosmia deafness hypogonadism syndrome
— Alopecia areata

— Alopecia congenita keratosis palmoplantaris
— Alopecia contractures dwarfism mental retardation
— Alopecia epilepsy oligophrenia syndrome of Moynahan
— Alopecia hypogonadism extrapyramidal disorder
— Alopecia immunodeficiency
— Alopecia macular degeneration growth retardation
— Alopecia mental retardation hypogonadism
— Alopecia mental retardation syndrome
— Alopecia totalis
— Alopecia universalis onychodystrophy vitiligo
— Alopecia universalis
— Alopecia, epilepsy, pyorrhea, mental subnormality
— Alopecia
— Alpers disease
— Alpha 1-antitrypsin deficiency
— Alpha-2 deficient collagen disease
— Alpha-ketoglutarate dehydrogenase deficiency
— Alpha-L-iduronidase deficiency
— Alpha-mannosidosis
— Alpha-sarcoglycanopathy
— Alpha-thalassemia
— Alpha-thalassemia-abnormal morphogenesis
— Alport syndrome macrothrombocytopenia
— Alport syndrome, dominant type
— Alport syndrome, recessive type
— Alport syndrome
— Alstrom's syndrome
— Alternating hemiplegia of childhood
— Alternating hemiplegia
— Aluminium lung
— Alveolar echinococcosis
— Alveolar soft part sarcoma
— Alveolitis, extrinsic allergic
— Alves Dos Santos Castello syndrome
— Alzheimer's disease
— Alzheimer disease, familial
— Amathophobia
— Amaurosis
— Amaurosis congenita of Leber, type 1
— Amaurosis congenita of Leber, type 2

— Amaurosis congenita of Leber
— Amaurosis hypertrichosis
— Amblyopia
— Ambral syndrome
— Ambras syndrome
— Amegakaryocytic thrombocytopenia
— Amelia cleft lip palate hydrocephalus iris coloboma
— Amelia facial dysmorphism
— Amelia X linked
— Amelogenesis Imperfecta hypomaturation type
— Amelogenesis imperfecta local hypoplastic form
— Amelogenesis imperfecta nephrocalcinosis
— Amelogenesis imperfecta
— Ameloonychohypohidrotic syndrome
— Amenorrhea
— American trypanosomiasis
— Aminoacidopathies
— Aminoaciduria
— Aminopterin antenatal infection
— Aminopterin like syndrome without aminopterin
— Amniotic bands
— Amoebiasis due to Entamoeba histolytica
— Amoebiasis due to free-living amoebae
— Amoebiasis or Amebiasis
— Ampola syndrome
— Amychophobia
— Amylo-1,6-glucosidase deficiency
— Amyloid angiopathy
— Amyloid Neuropathies, Familial
— Amyloid polyneuropathy, transthyretin related
— Amyloidosis of gingiva and conjunctiva mental retardation
— Amyloidosis, Familial
— Amyloidosis
— Amylopectinosis
— Amyoplasia mandibulofacial dysostosis
— Amyoplasia
— Amyotonia congenita
— Amyotrophic lateral sclerosis
— Anablephobia
— Anaphylaxis

— Anaplastic thyroid cancer
— Andersen's disease
— Andre syndrome
— Androgen insensitivity syndrome (AIS)
— Anemia sideroblastic spinocerebellar ataxia
— Anemia, Diamond-Blackfan
— Anemia, Hypoplastic, Congenital
— Anemia, Pernicious
— Anemia, Sideroblastic
— Anemia
— Anencephaly spina bifida X linked
— Anencephaly
— Aneurysm of sinus of Valsalva
— Aneurysm, intracranial berry
— Aneurysm
— Angel shaped phalangoepiphyseal dysplasia
— Angelman syndrome
— Angiofollicular ganglionic hyperplasia
— Angiofollicular lymph hyperplasia
— Angioimmunoblastic lymphadenopathy with dysproteinemia
— Angiokeratoma mental retardation coarse face
— Angiolipoma
— Angioma hereditary neurocutaneous
— Angiomatosis encephalotrigeminal
— Angiomatosis leptomeningeal capillary - venous
— Angiomatosis systemic cystic Seip syndrome
— Angiomyomatous Hamartoma
— Angioneurotic edema hereditary due to C1 esterase deficiency
— Angiosarcoma of the liver
— Angiosarcoma of the scalp
— Angiostrongyliasis
— Angiotensin renin aldosterone hypertension
— Anguillulosis
— Aniridia absent patella
— Aniridia ataxia renal agenesis psychomotor retardation
— Aniridia cerebellar ataxia mental deficiency
— Aniridia mental retardation syndrome
— Aniridia ptosis mental retardation obesity familial
— Aniridia renal agenesis psychomotor retardation
— Aniridia type 2

— Aniridia, sporadic
— Aniridia
— Anisakiasis
— Ankle defects short stature
— Ankyloblepharon ectodermal defects cleft lip palate
— Ankyloblepharon filiforme adnatum cleft palate
— Ankyloblepharon filiforme imperforate anus
— Ankyloglossia heterochromia clasped thumbs
— Ankylosing spondylarthritis
— Ankylosing spondylitis
— Ankylosing vertebral hyperostosis with tylosis
— Ankylosis of teeth
— Ankylostomiasis
— Annular constricting bands
— Annular pancreas
— Annuloaortic ectasia
— Anodontia
— Anonychia ectrodactyly
— Anonychia microcephaly
— Anonychia onychodystrophy brachydactyly type B
— Anonychia onychodystrophy
— Anophthalia pulmonary hypoplasia
— Anophthalmia cleft lip palate hypothalamic disorder
— Anophthalmia cleft palate micrognathia
— Anophthalmia esophageal atresia cryptorchidism
— Anophthalmia megalocornea cardiopathy skeletal anomalies
— Anophthalmia microcephaly hypogonadism
— Anophthalmia plus syndrome
— Anophthalmia short stature obesity
— Anophthalmia Waardenburg syndrome
— Anophthalmos with limb anomalies
— Anophthalmos, clinical
— Anorchia
— Anorchidism
— Anorectal anomalies
— Ano-rectal atresia
— Anorexia nervosa
— Anosmia
— Anotia facial palsy cardiac defect
— Anotia

— Ansell Bywaters Elderking syndrome
— Anterior horn disease
— Anterior pituitary insufficiency, familial
— Anthrax
— Anti-factor VIII autoimmunization
— Antigen-peptide-transporter 2 deficiency
— Anti-HLA hyperimmunization
— Antihypertensive drugs antenatal infection
— Antinolo Nieto Borrego syndrome
— Aplasia cutis autosomal recessive
— Aplasia cutis congenita dominant
— Aplasia cutis congenita epibulbar dermoids
— Aplasia cutis congenita intestinal lymphangiectasia
— Aplasia cutis congenita of limbs recessive
— Aplasia cutis congenita recessive
— Aplasia cutis congenita
— Aplasia cutis myopia
— Aplasia/hypoplasia of pelvis, femur, fibula, and ulna with abnormal digits and nails
— Aplastic anemia
— Apo A-I deficiency
— Apolipoprotein C-II deficiency
— Apparent mineralocorticoid excess
— Appelt-Gerken-Lenz syndrome
— Appendicitis
— Apraxia manual
— Apraxia, Ideomotor
— Apraxia, ocular motor, Cogan type
— Apraxia
— Apudoma
— Aqueductal stenosis, X linked
— Arachindonic acid, absence of
— Arachnodactyly ataxia cataract aminoaciduria mental retardation
— Arachnodactyly mental retardation dysmorphism
— Arachnoid cysts
— Arachnoiditis
— Arakawa'sa syndrome II
— Arbovirosis
— Arc syndrome

— Aredyld syndrome
— AREDYLD
— Arginase deficiency
— Arginemia
— Argininosuccinate synthetase deficiency
— Argininosuccinic aciduria
— Argyria
— Arhinia choanal atresia microphthalmia
— Arnold Stickler Bourne syndrome
— Arnold-Chiari malformation
— Aromatase deficiency
— Aromatic amino acid decarboxylase deficiency
— Arrhinia
— Arrhythmogenic right ventricular dysplasia
— Arroyo Garcia Cimadevilla syndrome
— Arrythmogenic right ventricular dysplasia, familial
— Arterial calcification of infancy
— Arterial dysplasia
— Arterial tortuosity
— Arteriovenous malformation
— Arteritis
— Arthritis short stature deafness
— Arthritis, Juvenile
— Arthritis
— Arthrogryposis due to muscular dystrophy
— Arthrogryposis ectodermal dysplasia other anomalies
— Arthrogryposis epileptic seizures migrational brain disorder
— Arthrogryposis IUGR thoracic dystrophy
— Arthrogryposis like disorder
— Arthrogryposis like hand anomaly sensorineural
— Arthrogryposis multiplex congenita CNS calcification
— Arthrogryposis multiplex congenita distal
— Arthrogryposis multiplex congenita neurogenic type
— Arthrogryposis multiplex congenita pulmonary hypoplasia
— Arthrogryposis multiplex congenita whistling face
— Arthrogryposis multiplex congenita, distal type 1
— Arthrogryposis multiplex congenita, distal type 2
— Arthrogryposis multiplex congenita, distal, x-linked
— Arthrogryposis multiplex congenita
— Arthrogryposis ophthalmoplegia retinopathy

- Arthrogryposis renal dysfunction cholestasis syndrome
- Arthrogryposis spinal muscular atrophy
- Arthrogryposis
- Arylsulfatase A deficiency
- Asbestosis
- Ascariasis
- Ascher's Syndrome
- Aseptic meningitis
- Asherman's syndrome
- Aspartylglycosaminuria
- Aspergillosis
- Asphyxia neonatorum
- Asthenia
- Asthma
- Astrocytoma
- Asymmetric septal hypertrophy
- Ataxia telangiectasia variant V1
- Ataxia telangiectasia
- Ataxia, Marie's
- Atelosteogenesis, type II
- Athabaskan brain stem dysgenesis
- Atherosclerosis
- Athetosis
- Athlete's foot
- Atopic Dermatitis
- Atresia of small intestine
- Atrial myxoma, familial
- Atrial septal defect
- Atrioventricular fistula
- Atrioventricular septal defect
- Atrophoderma of Pierini and Pasini
- Atrophy
- ATR-X
- Attention Deficit Hyperactivity Disorder
- Attenuated FAP
- Atypical lipodystrophy
- Auditory Perceptual Disorder
- Aughton syndrome
- Ausems Wittebol Post Hennekam syndrome
- Autoimmune hemolytic anemia

— Autoimmune hepatitis
— Autoimmune peripheral neuropathy
— Autoimmune polyendocrinopathy syndrome, type I
— Autonomic dysfunction
— Autonomic nervous system diseases
— Axial mesodermal dysplasia spectrum
— Axial osteomalacia
— Axial osteosclerosis
— Ayazi syndrome

B

— Baber's syndrome
— Babesiosis
— Bacterial endocarditis
— Bacterial food poisoning
— Bacterial gastroenteritis
— Bacterial meningitis
— Bacterial pneumonia
— BAER
— Bagatelle Cassidy syndrome
— Bahemuka Brown syndrome
— Baker Vinters syndrome
— Baker-Winegard syndrome
— Balantidiasis
— Ballard syndrome
— Ballistophobia
— Balo disease
— Balo's concentric sclerosis
— Bamforth syndrome
— BANF acoustic neurinoma
— Bangstad syndrome
— Banki syndrome
— Bannayan-Zonana syndrome
— Banti's syndrome
— Bantu siderosis
— Baraitser Brett Piesowicz syndrome
— Baraitser Rodeck Garner syndrome
— Barnicoat Baraitser syndrome
— Barrett syndrome
— Barrow Fitzsimmons syndrome

— Barth syndrome
— Bartonella infections
— Bartsocas Papa syndrome
— Bartter syndrome, antenatal form
— Bartter syndrome, classic form
— Basal cell carcinoma
— Basal cell nevus anodontia abnormal bone mineralization
— Basal ganglia diseases
— Basan syndrome
— Basaran Yilmaz syndrome
— Basedow's coma
— Basilar artery migraines
— Basilar impression primary
— Bassoe syndrome
— Bathophobia
— Batrachophobia
— Battaglia Neri syndrome
— Batten disease
— Batten Turner muscular dystrophy
— Baughman syndrome
— Bazex-Dupre-Christol syndrome
— Bazopoulou Kyrkanidou syndrome
— B-cell lymphomas
— Bd syndrome
— Beals syndrome
— Beardwell syndrome
— Bébé Collodion syndrome
— Becker disease
— Becker's muscular dystrophy
— Becker's nevus
— Beemer Ertbruggen syndrome
— Beemer Langer syndrome
— Behcet syndrome
— Behr syndrome
— Behrens Baumann Dust syndrome
— Bejel
— Bellini Chiumello Rinoldi syndrome
— Bell's palsy
— Ben Ari Shuper Mimouni syndrome
— Benallegue Lacete syndrome

— Bencze syndrome
— Benign astrocytoma
— Benign autosomal dominant myopathy
— Benign congenital hypotonia
— Benign essential blepharospasm
— Benign essential tremor syndrome
— Benign familial hematuria
— Benign familial infantile convulsions
— Benign familial infantile epilepsy
— Benign fasciculation syndrome
— Benign lymphoma
— Benign mucosal pemphigoid
— Benign paroxysmal positional vertigo
— Bentham Driessen Hanveld syndrome
— Berardinelli-Seip congenital lipodystrophy
— Berdon syndrome
— Berger disease
— Beriberi
— Berlin Breakage syndrome
— Berry aneurysm, cirrhosis, pulmonary emphysema, and cerebral calcification
— Berylliosis
— Besnier-Boeck-Schaumann disease
— Beta ketothiolase deficiency
— Beta-galactosidase-1 deficiency
— Beta-mannosidosis
— Beta-sarcoglycanopathy
— Beta-thalassemia major anemia
— Beta-thalassemia (gene promoter involvement)
— Bethlem myopathy
— Bhaskar Jagannathan syndrome
— Bibliophobia
— Bickel Fanconi glycogenosis
— Bicuspid aortic valve
— Bidirectional tachycardia
— Biemond syndrome type 1
— Biemond syndrome type 2
— Biemond syndrome
— Biermer disease
— Bifid nose dominant

— Bilateral renal agenesis dominant type
— Bilateral renal agenesis
— Biliary atresia, extrahepatic
— Biliary atresia, intrahepatic, non syndromic form
— Biliary atresia, intrahepatic, syndromic form
— Biliary atresia
— Biliary cirrhosis
— Biliary hypoplasia
— Biliary malformation renal tubular insufficiency
— Biliary tract cancer
— Billard Toutain Maheut syndrome
— Billet Bear syndrome
— Bindewald Ulmer Muller syndrome
— Binswanger's disease
— Bipolar disorder
— Biotinidase deficiency
— Bird headed dwarfism Montreal type
— Birdshot chorioretinopathy
— Birt-Hogg-Dube syndrome
— Bixler Christian Gorlin syndrome
— Bjornstad syndrome
— Bladder neoplasm
— Blaichman syndrome
— Blastoma
— Blastomycosis
— Blepharitis
— Blepharo cheilo dontic syndrome
— Blepharo facio skeletal syndrome
— Blepharo naso facial syndrome Van maldergem type
— Blepharonasofacial malformation syndrome
— Blepharophimosis nasal groove growth retardation
— Blepharophimosis ptosis esotropia syndactyly short
— Blepharophimosis ptosis syndactyly mental retardation
— Blepharophimosis syndrome Ohdo type
— Blepharophimosis, ptosis, epicanthus inversus
— Blepharophimosis
— Blepharoptosis aortic anomaly
— Blepharoptosis cleft palate ectrodactyly dental anomalies
— Blepharoptosis myopia ectopia lentis
— Blepharospasm

— Blethen Wenick Hawkins syndrome
— Blomstrand syndrome
— Blood Coagulation Disorders, Inherited
— Blood platelet disorders
— Blood vessel disorder
— Bloom syndrome
— Blount's disease
— Blue cone monochromatism
— Blue diaper syndrome
— Blue rubber bleb nevus
— BOD syndrome
— Boder syndrome
— Body dysmorphic disorder
— Boil
— Bone development disorder
— Bone dysplasia Azouz type
— Bone dysplasia corpus callosum agenesis
— Bone dysplasia lethal Holmgren type
— Bone dysplasia Moore type
— Bone fragility craniosynostosis proptosis hydrocephalus
— Bone marrow failure neurologic abnormalities
— Bone marrow failure
— Bone neoplasms
— Bone tumor (generic term)
— Bonneau-Beaumont syndrome
— Bonneman Meinecke Reich syndrome
— Bonnemann Meinecke syndrome
— Bonnevie Ullrich Turner syndrome
— Book syndrome
— Boomerang dysplasia
— Booth Haworth Dilling syndrome
— BOR syndrome
— Borjeson Syndrome
— Bork Stender Schmidt syndrome
— Borreliosis
— Borrone Di Rocco Crovato syndrome
— Boscherini Galasso Manca Bitti syndrome
— Bosma Henkin Christiansen syndrome
— Bothriocephalosis
— Botulism

— Boucher Neuhauser syndrome
— Boudhina Yedes Khiari syndrome
— Bourneville's disease or Bourneville-Pringle disease
— Bowen syndrome
— Bowen-Conradi syndrome
— Bowenoid papulosis
— Bowen's disease
— Bowing congenital short bones
— Bowing of long bones congenital
— Boylan Dew Greco syndrome
— Brachioskeletogenital syndrome
— Brachman-de Lange syndrome
— Brachycephalofrontonasal dysplasia
— Brachycephaly deafness cataract mental retardation
— Brachydactylous dwarfism Mseleni type
— Brachydactyly
— Brachydactyly absence of distal phalanges
— Brachydactyly anonychia
— Brachydactyly clinodactyly
— Brachydactyly dwarfism mental retardation
— Brachydactyly elbow wrist dysplasia
— Brachydactyly hypertension
— Brachydactyly long thumb type
— Brachydactyly mesomelia mental retardation heart defects
— Brachydactyly nystagmus cerebellar ataxia
— Brachydactyly preaxial hallux varus
— Brachydactyly scoliosis carpal fusion
— Brachydactyly small stature face anomalies
— Brachydactyly Smorgasbord type
— Brachydactyly tibial hypoplasia
— Brachydactyly type a1
— Brachydactyly type a2
— Brachydactyly type a3
— Brachydactyly type A5 nail dysplasia
— Brachydactyly type a6
— Brachydactyly type a7
— Brachydactyly type B
— Brachydactyly type C
— Brachydactyly type e
— Brachydactyly types b and e combined

— Brachymesomelia renal syndrome
— Brachymesophalangy 2 and 5
— Brachymesophalangy mesomelic short limbs osseous anomalies
— Brachymesophalangy type 2
— Brachymetapody anodontia hypotrichosis albinoidism
— Brachymorphism onychodysplasia dysphalangism syndrome
— Brachyolmia recessive Hobaek type
— Brachyolmia
— Brachytelephalangy characteristic facies Kallmann
— Braddock Carey syndrome
— Braddock Jones Superneau syndrome
— Bradykinesia
— Brain cavernous angioma
— Brain Neoplasms
— Brain Stem Neoplasms
— Branchial arch defects
— Branchial arch syndrome X linked
— Branchio oculo facial syndrome Hing type
— Branchio-oculo-facial syndrome
— Branchiootorenal syndrome
— Breast and ovarian cancer
— Breast cancer, familial
— Bright's disease
— Brittle bone disease
— Brittle bone syndrome lethal type
— Brittle cornea syndrome
— Broad beta disease
— Broad-betalipoproteinemia
— Bromidrosiphobia
— Bronchiectasis
— Bronchiectasis oligospermia
— Bronchiolitis obliterans with obstructive pulmonary disease
— Bronchiolotis obliterans organizing pneumonia (BOOP)
— Bronchitis, Chronic
— Bronchogenic cyst
— Bronchopulmonary amyloidosis
— Bronchopulmonary dysplasia
— Brown syndrome
— Brown-Sequard syndrome
— Brucellosis

— Bruck syndrome
— Brugada syndrome
— Brunoni syndrome
— Bruton type agammaglobulinemia
— Bruyn Scheltens syndrome
— Bubonic plague
— Budd-Chiari syndrome
— Buerger's disease
— Bulbospinal amyotrophy, X-linked
— Bulimia nervosa
— Bull Nixon syndrome
— Bullous dystrophy macular type
— Bullous ichtyosiform erythroderma congenita
— Bullous pemphigoid
— Buntinx Lormans Martin syndrome
— Burkitt's lymphoma
— Burn Goodship syndrome
— Burnett Schwartz Berberian syndrome
— Burning mouth syndrome- Type 3
— Burning mouth syndrome
— Buschke Ollendorff syndrome
— Bustos Simosa Pinto Cisternas syndrome
— Buttiens Fryns syndrome
— Butyrylcholinesterase deficiency
— Byssinosis

C

— C syndrome
— C1 esterase deficiency (angioedema)
— Cacchi-Ricci disease
— CACH syndrome
— Cacophobia
— Cafe au lait spots syndrome
— Caffey disease
— CAHMR syndrome
— Calcinosis cutis (see also CREST syndrome)
— Calciphylaxis
— Calculi
— Calderon Gonzalez Cantu syndrome
— Calloso genital dysplasia

— Callus disease
— Calpainopathy
— Calvarial hyperostosis
— Camera Marugo -Cohen syndrome
— Camfak syndrome
— Campomelia Cumming type
— Camptobrachydactyly
— Camptocormism
— Camptodactyly fibrous tissue hyperplasia skeletal dysplasia
— Camptodactyly joint contractures facial skeletal dysplasia
— Camptodactyly overgrowth unusual facies
— Camptodactyly syndrome Guadalajara type 1
— Camptodactyly syndrome Guadalajara type 2
— Camptodactyly taurinuria
— Camptodactyly vertebral fusion
— Camptomelic syndrome
— Campylobacter infection
— Camurati Engelmann disease
— Canavan leukodystrophy
— Cancer
— Candidiasis familial chronic
— Candidiasis
— Canga's bead symptom
— Canine distemper
— Cantalamessa Baldini Ambrosi syndrome
— Cantu Sanchez Corona Fragoso syndrome
— Cantu Sanchez Corona Garcia syndrome
— Cantu Sanchez Corona Hernandes syndrome
— Capillary leak syndrome with monoclonal gammopathy
— Capillary venous leptomeningeal angiomatosis
— Caplan's syndrome
— Capos syndrome
— Caratolo Cilio Pessagno syndrome
— Carbamoyl phosphate synthetase deficiency
— Carbamoyl-phosphate synthase I deficiency disease (ornithine carbamoyl phosphate deficiency)
— Carbohydrate deficient glycoprotein syndrome
— Carbon baby syndrome
— Carbonic anhydrase II deficiency
— Carcinoid syndrome

- Carcinoma of the vocal tract
- Carcinoma, squamous cell of head and neck
- Carcinoma, squamous cell
- Carcinophobia
- Cardiac amyloidosis
- Cardiac and laterality defects
- Cardiac arrest
- Cardiac conduction defect, familial
- Cardiac diverticulum
- Cardiac hydatid cysts with intracavitary expansion
- Cardiac malformation
- Cardiac tamponade
- Cardiac valvular dysplasia, X-linked
- Cardioauditory syndrome of Sanchez- Cascos
- Cardioauditory syndrome
- Cardiofacial syndrome short limbs
- Cardiofaciocutaneous syndrome
- Cardiogenital syndrome
- Cardiomelic syndrome Stratton Koehler type
- Cardiomyopathy:
    - Arrhythmogenic right ventricular cardiomyopathy
    - Cardiomyopathic lentiginosis
    - Cardiomyopathy cataract hip spine disease
    - Cardiomyopathy diabetes deafness
    - Dilated cardiomyopathy: Cardiomyopathy dilated with conduction defect type 1, Cardiomyopathy dilated with conduction defect type 2, Cardiomyopathy, familial dilated
    - Cardiomyopathy due to anthracyclines
    - Cardiomyopathy hearing loss type t RNA lysine gene mutation
    - Hypertrophic cardiomyopathy: familial
    - Cardiomyopathy hypogonadism metabolic anomalies
    - Cardiomyopathy spherocytosis
    - Cardiomyopathy, fatal fetal, due to myocardial calcification
    - Cardiomyopathy, X linked, fatal infantile
    - Restrictive cardiomyopathy
- Cardiophobia
- Cardioskeletal myopathy-neutropenia

— Cardiospasm
— Carey Fineman Ziter syndrome
— Carnevale Canun Mendoza syndrome
— Carnevale Hernandez Castillo syndrome
— Carnevale Krajewska Fischetto syndrome
— Carney syndrome
— Carnitine palmitoyl transferase 1 deficiency
— Carnitine palmitoyl transferase 2 deficiency
— Carnitine palmitoyl transferase deficiency
— Carnitine transporter deficiency
— Carnitine-acylcarnitine translocase deficiency
— Carnophobia
— Carnosinase deficiency
— Carnosinemia
— Caroli disease
— Carotenemia
— Carotid artery dissection
— Carpal deformity migrognathia microstomia
— Carpal tunnel syndrome
— Carpenter Hunter type
— Carpenter syndrome
— Carpo tarsal osteolysis recessive
— Carpotarsal osteochondromatosis
— Carrington syndrome
— Cartilage-hair hypoplasia
— Cartilage hair hypoplasia like syndrome
— Cartilaginous neoplasms
— Cartwright Nelson Fryns syndrome
— Cassia Stocco Dos Santos syndrome
— Castleman's disease
— Castro Gago Pombo Novo syndrome
— Cat cry syndrome - see Cri du chat
— Cat Eye syndrome
— Cat Rodrigues syndrome
— Cat-scratch disease
— Catagelophobia
— Catapedaphobia
— Cataract,congenital ichthyosis
— Cataract aberrant oral frenula growth retardation
— Cataract anterior polar dominant

— Cataract ataxia deafness
— Cataract cardiomyopathy
— Cataract congenital autosomal dominant
— Cataract congenital dominant non nuclear
— Cataract congenital Volkmann type
— Cataract congenital with microphthalmia
— Cataract dental syndrome
— Cataract Hutterite type
— Cataract hypertrichosis mental retardation
— Cataract mental retardation hypogonadism
— Cataract microcornea syndrome
— Cataract microphthalmia septal defect
— Cataract skeletal anomalies
— Cataract, alopecia, sclerodactyly
— Cataract, congenital, with microcornea or slight microphthalmia
— Cataract, total congenital
— Cataract-glaucoma
— CATCH 22 syndrome
— Catecholamine hypertension
— Catel Manzke syndrome
— Caudal appendage deafness
— Caudal duplication
— Caudal regression syndrome
— Causalgia
— Cavernous hemangioma
— Cavernous lymphangioma
— Cavernous sinus thrombosis
— Cayler syndrome
— CCA syndrome
— Ccge syndrome
— CCHS
— CDG syndrome type 1A
— CDG syndrome type 1B
— CDG syndrome type 1C
— CDG syndrome type 2
— CDG syndrome type 3
— CDG syndrome type 4
— CDG syndrome
— CDK4 linked melanoma
— Cecato De lima Pinheiro syndrome

— Celiac disease epilepsy occipital calcifications
— Celiac sprue
— Cenani Lenz syndactylism
— Cennamo Gangemi syndrome
— Central core disease
— Central diabetes insipidus
— Central nervous system protozoal infections
— Central serous chorioretinopathy
— Central type neurofibromatosis
— Centromeric instability immunodeficiency syndrome
— Centronuclear myopathy
— Centrotemporal epilepsy
— Cephalopolysyndactyly
— Ceramidase deficiency
— Ceramide trihexosidosis
— Ceraunophobia
— Cerebellar agenesis
— Cerebellar ataxia areflexia pes cavus optic atrophy
— Cerebellar ataxia ectodermal dysplasia
— Cerebellar ataxia infantile with progressive external ophthalmoplegia
— Cerebellar ataxia, dominant pure
— Cerebellar ataxia
— Cerebellar degeneration, subacute
— Cerebellar degeneration
— Cerebellar hypoplasia endosteal sclerosis
— Cerebellar hypoplasia tapetoretinal degeneration
— Cerebellar hypoplasia
— Cerebellar parenchymal degeneration
— Cerebelloolivary atrophy
— Cerebelloparenchymal disorder 3
— Cerebellum agenesis hydrocephaly
— Cerebral Amyloid Angiopathy, Familial
— Cerebral amyloid angiopathy
— Cerebral aneurysm
— Cerebral autosomal dominant arteriopathy with subcortical infarcts and leukoencephalopathy
— Cerebral calcification cerebellar hypoplasia
— Cerebral calcifications opalescent teeth phosphaturia
— Cerebral cavernous malformation

— Cerebral cavernous malformations
— Cerebral gigantism jaw cysts
— Cerebral gigantism
— Cerebral hypoxia
— Cerebral malformations hypertrichosis claw hands
— Cerebral palsy
— Cerebral thrombosis -
— Cerebral ventricle neoplasm
— Cerebro facio articular syndrome
— Cerebro facio thoracic dysplasia
— Cerebro oculo dento auriculo skeletal syndrome
— Cerebro oculo genital syndrome
— Cerebro oculo skeleto renal syndrome
— Cerebro reno digital syndrome
— Cerebroarthrodigital syndrome
— Cerebro-costo-mandibular syndrome
— Cerebro-oculo-facio-skeletal syndrome
— Cerebroretinal vasculopathy
— Ceroid lipofuscinois, neuronal 1, infantile
— Ceroid lipofuscinois, neuronal 2, late infantile
— Ceroid lipofuscinois, neuronal 3, juvenile
— Ceroid lipofuscinois, neuronal 4, adult type
— Ceroid lipofuscinois, neuronal 5, late infantile
— Ceroid lipofuscinois, neuronal 6, late infantile
— Ceroid lipofuscinois, neuronal
— Ceroid lipofuscinosis, neuronal 4
— Cervical cancer
— Cervical hypertrichosis neuropathy
— Cervical hypertrichosis peripheral neuropathy
— Cervical ribs sprengel anomaly polydactyly
— Cervical vertebral fusion
— Cervicooculoacoustic syndrome
— Chagas disease
— Chalazion
— Chanarin disease
— Chanarin Dorfman syndrome ichthyosis
— Chancroid
— Chandler's syndrome
— Chands syndrome
— Chang Davidson Carlson syndrome

— Chaotic atrial tachycardia
— Char syndrome
— Charcot disease
— Charcot Marie tooth disease deafness dominant type
— Charcot Marie tooth disease deafness mental retardation
— Charcot Marie Tooth disease deafness recessive type
— Charcot Marie Tooth type 1 aplasia cutis congenita
— Charcot-Marie-Tooth disease type 1A
— Charcot-Marie-Tooth disease type 1B
— Charcot-Marie-Tooth disease type 1C
— Charcot-Marie-Tooth disease type 2A
— Charcot-Marie-Tooth disease type 2B1
— Charcot-Marie-Tooth disease type 2B2
— Charcot-Marie-Tooth disease type 2C
— Charcot-Marie-Tooth disease type 2D
— Charcot-Marie-Tooth disease type 4A
— Charcot-Marie-Tooth disease type 4B
— Charcot-Marie-Tooth disease with ptosis and parkinsonism
— Charcot-Marie-Tooth disease, intermediate form
— Charcot-Marie-Tooth disease, neuronal, type A
— Charcot-Marie-Tooth disease, neuronal, type B
— Charcot-Marie-Tooth disease, neuronal, type D
— Charcot-Marie-Tooth disease, X-linked type 2, recessive
— Charcot-Marie-Tooth disease, X-linked type 3, recessive
— Charcot-Marie-Tooth disease
— Charcot-Marie-Tooth peroneal muscular atrophy, X-linked
— CHARGE Association
— Charles' Disease
— Charlie M syndrome
— Chavany-Brunhes syndrome
— Chediak-Higashi syndrome
— Cheilitis glandularis
— Chemke Oliver Mallek syndrome
— Chemodectoma
— Chemophobia
— Chen Kung Ho Kaufman Mcalister syndrome
— Cherubism
— Chiari type 1 malformation
— Chiari-Frommel syndrome
— Chickenpox

— Chikungunya
— CHILD syndrome ichthyosis
— Childhood disintegrative disorder
— Childhood pustular psoriasis
— Chimerism
— [[Chinese restuarant syndrome
— Chitayat Haj Chahine syndrome
— Chitayat Meunier Hodgkinson syndrome
— Chitayat Moore Del Bigio syndrome
— Chitty Hall Baraitser syndrome
— Chitty Hall Webb syndrome
— Chlamydia trachomatis
— Chlamydia
— Chlamydial and Gonococcal Conjunctivitis
— Choanal atresia deafness cardiac defects dysmorphia
— Cholangiocarcinoma
— Cholangitis, primary sclerosing
— Cholecystitis
— Choledochal cyst, hand malformation
— Cholelithiasis
— Cholemia, familial
— Cholera
— Cholerophobia
— Cholestasis pigmentary retinopathy cleft palate
— Cholestasis, progressive familial intrahepatic 1
— Cholestasis, progressive familial intrahepatic 2
— Cholestasis, progressive familial intrahepatic 3
— Cholestasis, progressive familial intrahepatic
— Cholestasis
— Cholestatic jaundice renal tubular insufficiency
— Cholesterol ester storage disease
— Cholesterol esterification disorder
— Cholesterol pneumonia
— Chondroblastoma
— Chondrocalcinosis familial articular
— Chondrocalcinosis
— Chondrodysplasia lethal recessive
— Chondrodysplasia pseudohermaphrodism syndrome
— Chondrodysplasia punctata 1, x-linked recessive
— Chondrodysplasia punctata with steroid sulfatase deficiency

— Chondrodysplasia punctata, brachytelephalangic
— Chondrodysplasia punctata, Sheffield type
— Chondrodysplasia punctata
— Chondrodysplasia situs inversus imperforate anus polydactyly
— Chondrodysplasia, Grebe type
— Chondrodystrophy
— Chondroectodermal dysplasia
— Chondroma (benign)
— Chondromalacia
— Chondromatosis (benign)
— Chondrosarcoma (malignant)
— Chondrysplasia punctata, humero-metacarpal type
— Chordoma
— Chorea acanthocytosis
— Chorea familial benign
— Chorea minor
— Chorea
— Choreoacanthocytosis amyotrophic
— Choreoathetosis familial paroxysmal
— Choriocarcinoma
— Chorioretinitis
— Chorioretinopathy dominant form microcephaly
— Choroid plexus cyst
— Choroid Plexus neoplasms
— Choroidal atrophy alopecia
— Choroideremia hypopituitarism
— Choroideremia
— Choroiditis, serpiginous
— Choroiditis
— Choroido cerebral calcification syndrome infantile
— Christian Demyer Franken syndrome
— Christian Johnson Angenieta syndrome
— Christian syndrome
— Christianson Fourie syndrome
— Christmas disease
— Chromhidrosis
— Chromomycosis
— Chromophobe renal carcinoma
— Chromophobia
— Chromosomal triplication

— Chromosomes 1 and 2, monosomy 2q duplication 1p
— Chronic berylliosis
— Chronic demyelinizing neuropathy with IgM monoclonal
— Chronic erosive gastritis
— Chronic fatigue immune dysfunction syndrome
— Chronic fatigue syndrome
— Chronic granulomatous disease
— Chronic hiccup
— Chronic inflammatory demyelinating polyneuropathy
— Chronic lymphocytic leukemia
— Chronic mountain sickness
— Chronic myelogenous leukemia
— Chronic myelomonocytic leukemia
— Chronic necrotizing vasculitis
— Chronic neutropenia
— Chronic obstructive pulmonary disease
— Chronic polyradiculoneuritis
— Chronic recurrent multifocal osteomyelitis
— Chronic renal failure
— Chronic spasmodic dysphonia
— Chronic, infantile, neurological, cutaneous, articular syndrome
— Chudley Lowry Hoar syndrome
— Chudley Rozdilsky syndrome
— Chudley-Mccullough syndrome
— Churg-Strauss syndrome
— Chylous ascites
— Cicatricial pemphigoid
— Ciguatera fish poisoning
— Ciliary discoordination, due to random ciliary orientation
— Ciliary dyskinesia, due to transposition of ciliary microtubules
— Ciliary dyskinesia-bronchiectasis
— Cilliers Beighton syndrome
— Cinchonism
— Circumscribed cutaneous aplasia of the vertex
— Circumscribed disseminated keratosis Jadassohn Lew type
— Citrullinemia
— Clarkson disease
— Clayton Smith Donnai syndrome
— Cleft hand absent tibia
— Cleft lip and palate malrotation cardiopathy

— Cleft lip and/or palate with mucous cysts of lower
— Cleft lip palate abnormal thumbs microcephaly
— Cleft lip palate deafness sacral lipoma
— Cleft lip palate dysmorphism Kumar type
— Cleft lip palate ectrodactyly
— Cleft lip palate incisor and finger anomalies
— Cleft lip palate mental retardation corneal opacity
— Cleft lip palate oligodontia syndactyly pili torti
— Cleft lip palate pituitary deficiency
— Cleft lip palate-tetraphocomelia
— Cleft lip with or without cleft palate
— Cleft lip
— Cleft lower lip cleft lateral canthi chorioretinal
— Cleft palate cardiac defect ectrodactyly
— Cleft palate colobomata radial synostosis deafness
— Cleft palate heart disease polydactyly absent tibia
— Cleft palate lateral synechia syndrome
— Cleft palate short stature vertebral anomalies
— Cleft palate stapes fixation oligodontia
— Cleft palate X linked
— Cleft palate
— Cleft tongue syndrome
— Cleft upper lip median cutaneous polyps
— Clefting ectropion conical teeth
— Cleidocranial dysplasia micrognathia absent thumbs
— Cleidocranial dysplasia
— Cleisiophobia
— Climacophobia
— Clinophobia
— Cloacal exstrophy
— Clouston syndrome
— Cloverleaf skull bone dysplasia
— Cloverleaf skull micromelia thoracic dysplasia
— Clubfoot
— Cluster headache
— CMV antenatal infection
— Coach syndrome
— Coal worker's pneumoconiosis
— Coarctation of aorta dominant
— Coarse face hypotonia constipation

— Coats disease
— Cocaine antenatal infection
— Cocaine fetopathy
— Coccidioidomycosis
— Cochin Jewish Disorder
— Cockayne syndrome type 1
— Cockayne syndrome type 2
— Cockayne syndrome type 3
— Cockayne's syndrome
— Codas syndrome
— Coenzyme Q cytochrome c reductase deficiency of
— Coffin-Lowry syndrome
— Coffin-Siris syndrome
— COFS syndrome
— Cogan-Reese syndrome
— Cogan syndrome
— Cohen Hayden syndrome
— Cohen Lockood Wyborney syndrome
— Cohen syndrome
— Colavita Kozlowski syndrome
— Cold agglutination syndrome
— Cold agglutinin disease
— Cold antibody hemolytic anemia
— Cold contact urticaria
— Cold urticaria
— Cole carpenter syndrome
— Coleman Randall syndrome
— Colitis
— Collagen disorder
— Collagenous colitis
— Collins Pope syndrome
— Collins Sakati syndrome
— Coloboma chorioretinal cerebellar vermis aplasia
— Coloboma hair abnormality
— Coloboma of choroid and retina
— Coloboma of eye lens
— Coloboma of iris
— Coloboma of lens ala nasi
— Coloboma of macula type B brachydactyly
— Coloboma of macula

— Coloboma of optic nerve
— Coloboma of optic papilla
— Coloboma porencephaly hydronephrosis
— Coloboma uveal with cleft lip palate and mental retardation
— Coloboma, ocular
— Colobomata unilobar lung heart defect
— Colobomatous microphthalmia heart disease hearing
— Colobomatous microphthalmia
— Colon cancer, familial nonpolyposis
— Colonic atresia
— Colonic malakoplakia
— Color blindness
— Colorado tick fever
— Colver Steer Godman syndrome
— Combarros Calleja Leno syndrome
— Combined hyperlipidemia, familial
— Common cold
— Common mesentery
— Common variable immunodeficiency
— Compartment syndrome
— Complement component 2 deficiency
— Complement component receptor 1
— Complete atrioventricular canal
— Condyloma
— Cone dystrophy
— Cone rod dystrophy amelogenesis imperfecta
— Cone rod dystrophy
— Cranioacrofacial syndrome
— Craniodiaphyseal dysplasia
— Craniodigital syndrome mental retardation
— Cranioectodermal dysplasia
— Craniofacial and osseous defects mental retardation
— Craniofacial and skeletal defects
— Craniofacial deafness hand syndrome
— Craniofacial dysostosis arthrogryposis progeroid appearance
— Craniofacial dysostosis
— Craniofacial dysynostosis
— Craniofaciocardioskeletal syndrome
— Craniofaciocervical osteoglyphic dysplasia
— Craniofrontonasal dysplasia

— Craniofrontonasal syndrome Teebi type
— Craniometaphyseal dysplasia dominant type
— Craniometaphyseal dysplasia recessive type
— Craniomicromelic syndrome
— Craniostenosis cataract
— Craniostenosis with congenital heart disease mental retardation
— Craniostenosis
— Craniosynostosis alopecia brain defect
— Craniosynostosis arthrogryposis cleft palate
— Craniosynostosis autosomal dominant
— Craniosynostosis cleft lip palate arthrogryposis
— Craniosynostosis contractures cleft
— Craniosynostosis exostoses nevus epibulbar dermoid
— Craniosynostosis fibular aplasia
— Craniosynostosis Fontaine type
— Craniosynostosis Maroteaux Fonfria type
— Craniosynostosis mental retardation clefting syndrome
— Craniosynostosis mental retardation heart defects
— Craniosynostosis Philadelphia type
— Craniosynostosis radial aplasia syndrome
— Craniosynostosis synostoses hypertensive nephropathy
— Craniosynostosis Warman type
— Craniosynostosis, sagittal, with Dandy-Walker malformation and hydrocephalus
— Craniosynostosis
— Craniotelencephalic dysplasia
— Crawfurd syndrome
— Creatine deficiency
— Creeping disease
— CREST syndrome
— Cretinism athyreotic
— Cretinism
— Creutzfeldt-Jakob disease
— Cri du chat
— Crigler-Najjar syndrome
— Crisponi syndrome
— Criss cross syndrome
— Criswick-Schepens syndrome
— Crohn's disease of the esophagus
— Crohn's disease

— Crome syndrome
— Cronkhite-Canada disease
— Crossed polydactyly type 1
— Crossed polysyndactyly
— Croup
— Crouzon syndrome
— Crouzonodermoskeletal syndrome
— Crow-Fukase syndrome
— Cryoglobulinemia
— Cryophobia
— Cryptococcosis
— Cryptogenic organized pneumopathy
— Cryptomicrotia brachydactyly syndrome excess fingers
— Cryptomicrotia brachydactyly syndrome
— Cryptophthalmos-syndactyly syndrome
— Cryptorchidism arachnodactyly mental retardation
— Cryroglobulinemia
— Crystal deposit disease
— Crystallophobia
— Culler Jones syndrome
— Curly hair ankyloblepharon nail dysplasia syndrome
— Currarino triad
— Curry Hall syndrome
— Curth-Macklin type ichthyosis hystrix
— Curtis Rogers Stevenson syndrome
— Cushing syndrome, familial
— Cushing's symphalangism
— Cushing's syndrome
— Cutaneous anthrax
— Cutaneous larva migrans
— Cutaneous lupus erythematosus
— Cutaneous photosensitivity colitis lethal
— Cutaneous T-cell lymphoma
— Cutaneous vascularitis
— Cutis Gyrata syndrome of Beare and Stevenson
— Cutis gyratum acanthosis nigricans craniosynostosis
— Cutis laxa, recessive
— Cutis laxa corneal clouding mental retardation
— Cutis laxa osteoporosis
— Cutis laxa with joint laxity and retarded development

— Cutis laxa, dominant type
— Cutis laxa, recessive type 1
— Cutis laxa, recessive type 2
— Cutis laxa
— Cutis marmorata telangiectatica congenita
— Cutis verticis gyrata mental deficiency
— Cutis verticis gyrata thyroid aplasia mental retardation
— Cutis verticis gyrata
— Cutler Bass Romshe syndrome
— Cyclic neutropenia
— Cyclic vomiting syndrome
— Cyclosporosis
— Cypress facial neuromusculoskeletal syndrome
— Cystathionine beta synthetase deficiency
— Cystic adenomatoid malformation of lung
— Cystic angiomatosis of bone, diffuse
— Cystic fibrosis gastritis megaloblastic anemia
— Cystic fibrosis
— Cystic hamartoma of lung and kidney
— Cystic hygroma lethal cleft palate
— Cystic hygroma
— Cystic medial necrosis of aorta
— Cystin transport, protein defect of
— Cystinosis
— Cystinuria
— Cystinuria-lysinuria
— Cytochrome C oxidase deficiency
— Cytomegalic inclusion disease
— Cytomegalovirus
— Cytoplasmic body myopathy
— Czeizel Losonci syndrome
— Czeizel syndrome

D

— D ercole syndrome
— Daentl Towsend Siegel syndrome
— Dahlberg Borer Newcomer syndrome
— Daish Hardman Lamont syndrome
— Dandy Walker facial hemangioma
— Dandy Walker malformation postaxial polydactyly

— Dandy Walker syndrome recessive form
— Dandy-walker malformation with mental retardation, basal ganglia disease, and seizures
— Dandy-walker malformation with mental retardation, macrocephaly, myopia, and brachytelephalangy
— Dandy-Walker syndrome
— Daneman Davy Mancer syndrome
— Darier's disease
— Davenport Donlan syndrome
— David syndrome
— Davis Lafer syndrome
— De Barsy syndrome
— De Hauwere Leroy Adriaenssens syndrome
— De Sanctis-Cacchione syndrome
— Deaf blind hypopigmentation
— Dehydratase deficiency
— Dejerine-Sottas disease
— Delayed membranous cranial ossification
— Delayed speech facial asymmetry strabismus ear lobe creases
— Deletion 6q16 q21
— Delleman Oorthuys syndrome
— Delta-1-pyrroline-5-carboxylate dehydrogenase deficiency
— Delta-sarcoglycanopathy
— Dementia progressive lipomembranous polycysta
— Dementia, familial British
— Dementophobia
— Demodicidosis
— Demonophobia
— Demyelinating disease
— Dendrophobia
— Dengue fever
— Dennis Cohen syndrome
— Dennis Fairhurst Moore syndrome
— Dent disease
— Dental aberrations steroid dehydrogenase deficienciency
— Dental fluorosis
— Dental tissue neoplasm
— Dentatorubral pallidoluysian atrophy
— Dentin dysplasia sclerotic bones
— Dentin dysplasia, coronal

— Dentin dysplasia, radicular
— Dentinogenesis imperfecta
— Dentophobia
— Depersonalization disorder
— Depression (clinical)
— Dercum's disease aka Adiposis dolorosa
— Der kaloustian Jarudi Khoury syndrome
— Der Kaloustian Mcintosh Silver syndrome
— Dermatitis herpetiformis
— Dermatocardioskeletal syndrome Boronne type
— Dermatographic urticaria
— Dermatofibroma
— Dermatoleukodystrophy
— Dermatomyositis
— Dermatoosteolysis Kirghizian type
— Dermatopathia pigmentosa reticularis
— Dermatophobia
— Dermatophytids
— Dermatophytosis
— Dermochondrocorneal dystrophy of François
— Dermoodontodysplasia
— Desbuquois syndrome
— Desmin related myopathy
— Desmoid disease
— Desmoid tumor
— Desmoplastic small round cell tumor
— Developmental delay hypotonia extremities hypertrophy
— Developmental dysphasia familial
— Devic syndrome
— Devriendt Legius Fryns syndrome
— Devriendt Vandenberghe Fryns syndrome
— Dexamethasone sensitive hypertension
— Dextrocardia with situs inversus
— Dextrocardia
— Dextrocardia-bronchiectasis-sinusitis
— D-glycerate dehydrogenase deficiency
— D-glycericacidemia
— Diabetes hypogonadism deafness mental retardation
— Diabetes insipidus
— Diabetes insipidus, diabetes mellitus, optic atrophy

— Diabetes insipidus, nephrogenic type 1
— Diabetes insipidus, nephrogenic type 2
— Diabetes insipidus, nephrogenic type 3
— Diabetes insipidus, nephrogenic, dominant type
— Diabetes insipidus, nephrogenic, recessive type
— Diabetes mellitus
— Diabetes mellitus, transient neonatal
— Diabetes persistent mullerian ducts
— Diabetes, insulin dependent
— Diabetic angiopathy
— Diabetic embryopathy
— Diabetic nephropathy
— Diabetic neuropathy
— Diamond Blackfan disease
— Diaphragmatic agenesia
— Diaphragmatic agenesis radial aplasia omphalocele
— Diaphragmatic defect limb deficiency skull defect
— Diaphragmatic hernia abnormal face limb
— Diaphragmatic hernia exomphalos corpus callosum agenesis
— Diaphragmatic hernia upper limb defects
— Diaphragmatic hernia, congenital
— Diarrhea chronic with villous atrophy
— Diarrhea polyendocrinopathy infections X linked
— Diastematomyelia
— Diastrophic dysplasia
— Dibasic aminoaciduria 2
— Dibasic aminoaciduria type 1
— Dicarboxylicaminoaciduria
— Die Smulders Droog Van Dijk syndrome
— Die Smulders Vles Fryns syndrome
— Diencephalic syndrome
— Dieterich's disease
— Diethylstilbestrol antenatal infection
— Diffuse idiopathic skeletal hyperostosis
— Diffuse leiomyomatosis with Alport syndrome
— Diffuse neonatal hemangiomatosis
— Diffuse palmoplantar keratoderma, Bothnian type
— Diffuse panbronchiolitis
— DiGeorge syndrome
— Digestive duplication

— Digitorenocerebral syndrome
— Dihydropteridine reductase deficiency
— Dihydropyrimidine dehydrogenase deficiency
— Dilated cardiomyopathy
— Dimitri Sturge Weber syndrome
— Dincsoy Salih Patel syndrome
— Dinno Shearer Weisskopf syndrome
— Dinophobia
— Diomedi Bernardi Placidi syndrome
— Dionisi Vici Sabetta Gambarara syndrome
— Diphallia
— Diphallus rachischisis imperforate anus
— Diphosphoglycerate mutase deficiency of erythrocyte
— Diphtheria
— Disaccharide intolerance iii
— Discoid lupus erythematosus
— Dislocation of the hip dysmorphism
— Disorder in the hormonal synthesis with or without goiter
— Disorganization syndrome
— Dissecting cellulitis of the scalp
— Dissociative amnesia
— Dissociative hysteria
— Dissociative fugue
— Dissociative identity disorder
— Distal arthrogryposis Moore Weaver type
— Distal myopathy Markesbery-Griggs type
— Distal myopathy with vocal cord weakness
— Distal myopathy, Nonaka type
— Distal myopathy
— Distal primary acidosis, familial
— Distemper
— Distichiasis heart congenital anomalies
— Distomatosis
— Diverticulitis
— Diverticulosis
— Dk phocomelia syndrome
— D-minus hemolytic uremic syndrome
— Dobrow syndrome
— Dominant cleft palate
— Dominant ichthyosis vulgaris

— Dominant zonular cataract
— Donnai Barrow syndrome
— Door syndrome
— Dopamine beta-hydroxylase deficiency
— DOPA-responsive dystonia
— Doraphobia
— Double cortex
— Double discordia
— Double fingernail of fifth finger
— Double outlet left ventricle
— Double outlet right ventricle
— Double tachycardia induced by catecholamines
— Double uterus-hemivagina-renal agenesis
— Downs Syndrome
— Doxorubicin-induced cardiomyopathy
— Doyne honeycomb retinal dystrophy
— D-plus hemolytic uremic syndrome
— Drachtman Weinblatt Sitarz syndrome
— Dracunculiasis
— Duane anomaly mental retardation
— Duane syndrome
— Dubin-Johnson syndrome
— Dubowitz syndrome
— Duchenne muscular dystrophy
— Duhring Brocq disease
— Duhring's disease
— Duker Weiss Siber syndrome
— Duodenal atresia tetralogy of Fallot
— Duodenal atresia
— Duplication of leg mirror foot
— Duplication of the thumb unilateral biphalangeal
— Duplication of urethra
— Dupont Sellier Chochillon syndrome
— Dupuytren subungual exostosis
— Dupuytren's contracture
— Dust-induced lung disease
— Dwarfism bluish sclerae
— Dwarfism deafness retinitis pigmentosa
— Dwarfism lethal type advanced bone age
— Dwarfism mental retardation eye abnormality

— Dwarfism short limb absent fibulas very short digits
— Dwarfism stiff joint ocular abnormalities
— Dwarfism syndesmodysplasic
— Dwarfism tall vertebrae
— Dwarfism thanatophoric
— Dwarfism thin bones multiple fractures
— Dwarfism
— Dyggve-Melchior-Clausen syndrome
— Dykes Markes Harper syndrome
— Dysautonomia (does not have to be familial) (Autonomic Nervous System Diseases)
— Dysbarism
— Dyschondrosteosis nephritis
— Dyschromatosis universalis
— Dysencephalia splachnocystica or Meckel Gruber
— Dysequilibrium syndrome
— Dyserythropoietic anemia, congenital type 1
— Dyserythropoietic anemia, congenital type 2
— Dyserythropoietic anemia, congenital type 3
— Dyserythropoietic anemia, congenital
— Dysferlinopathy
— Dysfibrinogenemia, familial
— Dysgerminoma
— Dysharmonic skeletal maturation muscular fiber disproportion
— Dyskeratosis congenita of Zinsser Cole Engman
— Dyskeratosis congenita
— Dyskeratosis follicularis
— Dyskinesia, drug induced
— Dyskinesia
— Dysmorphism abnormal vocalization mental retardation
— Dysmorphism cleft palate loose skin
— Dysmorphophobia
— Dysmyelination
— Dysosteosclerosis
— Dysostosis acral with facial and genital abnormalities
— Dysostosis peripheral
— Dysostosis Stanescu type
— Dysostosis
— Dysphasic dementia, hereditary
— Dysphonia, chronic spasmodic

— Dysplasia epiphysealis hemimelica
— Dysplasia
— Dysplastic cortical hyperostosis
— Dysplastic nevus syndrome
— Dysprothrombinemia
— Dysraphism cleft lip palate limb reduction defects
— Dyssegmental dysplasia glaucoma
— Dyssegmental dysplasia Silverman Handmaker type
— Dysthymia
— Dystonia musculorum deformans type 1
— Dystonia musculorum deformans type 2
— Dystonia musculorum deformans
— Dystonia progressive with diurnal variation
— Dystonia
— Dystrophia myotonica
— Dystrophic epidermolysis bullosa
— Dystrophinopathy
— Dystychiphobia

E

— EAF
— Eales disease
— Ear, patella, short stature syndrome
— Earlobes thickened conductive deafness
— Ebola hemorrhagic fever
— Ebstein's anomaly
— Eccentrochondrodysplasia
— Eccrine acrospiroma
— Eclampsia
— Ecp syndrome
— Ectodermal dysplasia absent dermatoglyphics
— Ectodermal dysplasia adrenal cyst
— Ectodermal dysplasia alopecia preaxial polydactyly
— Ectodermal dysplasia anhidrotic
— Ectodermal dysplasia arthrogryposis diabetes mellitus
— Ectodermal dysplasia Bartalos type
— Ectodermal dysplasia Berlin type
— Ectodermal dysplasia blindness
— Ectodermal dysplasia ectrodactyly macular dystrophy
— Ectodermal dysplasia hypohidrotic autosomal dominant

— Ectodermal dysplasia hypohidrotic hypothyroidism ciliary diskinesia
— Ectodermal dysplasia Margarita type
— Ectodermal dysplasia mental retardation CNS malformation
— Ectodermal dysplasia mental retardation syndactyly
— Ectodermal dysplasia neurosensory deafness
— Ectodermal dysplasia osteosclerosis
— Ectodermal dysplasia tricho odonto onychial type
— Ectodermal dysplasia, hydrotic
— Ectodermal dysplasia, hypohidrotic, autosomal recessive
— Ectodermal Dysplasia
— Ectodermal dysplasias
— Ectodermic dysplasia anhidrotic cleft lip
— Ectopia cordis
— Ectopia lentis isolated
— Ectopia pupillae
— Ectopic coarctation
— Ectopic ossification familial type
— Ectopic pregnancy
— Ectrodactyly cardiopathy dysmorphism
— Ectrodactyly cleft palate syndrome
— Ectrodactyly diaphragmatic hernia corpus callosum
— Ectrodactyly dominant form
— Ectrodactyly ectrodermal dysplasia
— Ectrodactyly polydactyly
— Ectrodactyly recessive form
— Ectrodactyly
— Ectrodactyly-ectodermal dysplasia-cleft lip/cleft palate
— Ectropion inferior cleft lip and or palate
— Edinburgh malformation syndrome
— Edwards Patton Dilly syndrome
— Edwards syndrome
— Eec syndrome without cleft lip palate
— Eec syndrome
— Eem syndrome
— Egg hypersensitivity
— Egg shaped pupils
— Ehlers-Danlos syndrome
— Ehrlichiosis
— Eijkman's syndrome

— Eiken syndrome
— Eisenmenger syndrome
— Eisoptrophobia
— Elattoproteus in context of NF
— Elective mutism
— Ectrodactyly-ectodermal dysplasia-cleft syndrome
— Electron transfer flavoprotein, deficiency of
— Electrophobia
— Elejalde syndrome
— Elephant man in context of NF
— Elephantiasis
— Elliott Ludman Teebi syndrome
— Ellis Yale Winter syndrome
— Ellis-Van Creveld syndrome
— Emerinopathy
— Emery Nelson syndrome
— Emery-Dreifuss muscular dystrophy, dominant type
— Emery-Dreifuss muscular dystrophy, X-linked
— Emery-Dreifuss muscular dystrophy
— Emetophobia
— Emphysema, congenital lobar
— Emphysema
— Emphysema-penoscrotal web-deafness-mental retardation
— Empty sella syndrome
— Enamel hypoplasia cataract hydrocephaly
— Encephalitis
— Encephalitis lethargica
— Encephalo cranio cutaneous lipomatosis
— Encephalocele anencephaly
— Encephalocele anterior
— Encephalocele frontal
— Encephalocele
— Encephalomyelitis, Myalgic
— Encephalomyelitis
— Encephalopathy intracerebral calcification retinal
— Encephalopathy progressive optic atrophy
— Encephalopathy subacute spongiform, Gerstmann-Stra
— Encephalopathy-basal ganglia-calcification
— Encephalophathy recurrent of childhood
— Encephalotrigeminal angiomatosis

- — Enchondromatosis (benign)
- — Enchondromatosis dwarfism deafness
- — Endocardial fibroelastosis
- — Endocarditis, infective
- — Endocarditis
- — Endocrinopathy
- — Epiphysealis hemimelica dysplasia
- — Epistaxiophobia
- — Epithelial-myoepithelial carcinoma
- — Epitheliopathy (APMPPE)
- — Epitheliopathy, acute posterior multifocal placoid
- — EPP (erythropoietic protoporphyria)
- — Epstein barr virus mononucleosis
- — Epstein syndrome
- — Equinophobia
- — Erb-Duchenne palsy
- — Erdheim disease
- — Erdheim-Chester syndrome
- — Ereuthrophobia
- — Ergophobia
- — Eronen Somer Gustafsson syndrome
- — Erosive pustular dermatosis of the scalp
- — Erysipelas
- — Erythema multiforme
- — Erythermalgia
- — Erythroblastopenia
- — Erythroderma desquamativa of Leiner
- — Erythroderma lethal congenital
- — Erythrokeratodermia ataxia
- — Erythrokeratodermia progressive symmetrica ichthyosis
- — Erythrokeratodermia symmetrica progressiva
- — Erythrokeratodermia variabilis ichthyosis
- — Erythrokeratodermia variabilis, Mendes da Costa type
- — Erythrokeratodermia with ataxia
- — Erythrokeratolysis hiemalis ichthyosis
- — Erythromelalgia
- — Erythroplakia
- — Erythropoietic protoporphyria
- — Escher Hirt syndrome
- — Esophageal atresia associated anomalies

— Esophageal atresia coloboma talipes
— Esophageal atresia
— Esophageal disorder
— Esophageal duodenal atresia abnormalities of hands
— Esophageal neoplasm
— Esophageal varices
— Esotropia
— Essential hypertension
— Essential iris atrophy
— Essential mixed cryoglobulinemia
— Essential thrombocytopenia
— Essential thrombocythemia - synonym of Essential thrombocytosis
— Essential thrombocytosis
— Esthesioneuroblastoma
— Ethylmalonic aciduria
— Ethylmalonic adipic aciduria
— Euhidrotic ectodermal dysplasia
— Eunuchoidism familial
— Euphobia
— Evan's syndrome
— Ewing's Sarcoma
— Exencephaly
— Exercise induced anaphylaxis
— Exfoliative dermatitis
— Exner syndrome
— Exogenous lipoid pneumonia
— Exomphalos-macroglossia-gigantism syndrome
— Exophthalmos
— Exostoses anetodermia brachydactyly type E
— Exostoses, multiple, type 1
— Exostoses, multiple, type 2
— Exostoses, multiple, type 3
— Exostoses, multiple
— Exostoses
— Experimental allergic encephalomyelitis
— Exploding head syndrome
— Exstrophy of the bladder
— Exstrophy of the bladder-epispadias
— Exudative retinopathy familial, autosomal dominant

— Exudative retinopathy familial, autosomal recessive
— Exudative retinopathy familial, X linked, recessive
— Exudative retinopathy, familial
— Extrapyramidal disorder
— Extrasystoles short stature hyperpigmentation microcephaly
— Eye defects arachnodactyly cardiopathy
— Eyebrows duplication syndactyly

F

— Fabry's disease
— Faces syndrome
— Facial asymmetry temporal seizures
— Facial clefting corpus callosum agenesis
— Facial dysmorphism macrocephaly myopia Dandy Walker type
— Facial dysmorphism shawl scrotum joint laxity syndrome
— Facial paralysis
— Facies unusual arthrogryposis advanced skeletal malformations
— Facio digito genital syndrome recessive form
— Facio skeletal genital syndrome Rippberger type
— Facio thoraco genital syndrome
— Faciocardiomelic dysplasia lethal
— Faciocardiorenal syndrome
— Faciooculoacousticorenal syndrome
— Facioscapulohumeral muscular dystrophy
— Factor II deficiency
— Factor V deficiency
— Factor V Leiden mutation
— Factor VII deficiency
— Factor VIII deficiency
— Factor X deficiency, congenital
— Factor X deficiency
— Factor XI deficiency, congenital
— Factor XIII deficiency, congenital
— Factor XIII deficiency
— Fahr's disease
— Fairbank disease
— Fallot tetralogy
— Familial Treacher Collins syndrome
— Familial veinous malformations
— Familial ventricular tachycardia

— Familial visceral myopathy
— Familial wilms tumor 2
— Fan death
— Fanconi anemia type 1
— Fanconi anemia type 2
— Fanconi anemia type 3
— Fanconi Bickel syndrome
— Fanconi ichthyosis dysmorphism
— Fanconi like syndrome
— Fanconi pancytopenia
— Fanconi syndrome
— Fanconi syndrome, renal, with nephrocalcinosis and renal stones
— Fanconi's anemia
— Fara Chlupackova syndrome
— Farber's disease
— Farmer's lung
— Fas deficiency
— Fascioliasis
— Fatal familial insomnia
— Fatty liver
— Faulk Epstein Jones syndrome
— Faye Petersen Ward Carey syndrome
— Fazio Londe syndrome
— Fealty syndrome
— Febrile seizure
— Fechtner syndrome
— Feigenbaum Bergeron Richardson syndrome
— Feigenbaum Bergeron syndrome
— Feingold Trainer syndrome
— Felty's Syndrome
— Female pseudohermaphrodism Genuardi type
— Female pseudohermaphroditism
— Femoral facial syndrome
— Femur bifid with monodactylous ectrodactyly
— Femur fibula ulna syndrome
— Fenton Wilkinson Toselano syndrome
— Ferlini Ragno Calzolari syndrome
— Fernhoff Blackston Oakley syndrome
— Ferrocalcinosis cerebro vascular
— Fetal acitretin syndrome

— Fetal akinesia syndrome X linked
— Fetal aminopterin syndrome
— Fetal and neonatal alloimmune thrombocytopenia
— Fetal antihypertensive drugs syndrome
— Fetal brain disruption sequence
— Fetal cytomegalovirus syndrome
— Fetal diethylstilbestrol syndrome
— Fetal edema
— Fetal enterovirus syndrome
— Fetal hydantoin syndrome
— Fetal indomethacin syndrome
— Fetal iodine syndrome
— Fetal left ventricular aneurysm
— Fetal methimazole syndrome
— Fetal methyl mercury syndrome
— Fetal minoxidil syndrome
— Fetal parainfluenza virus type 3 syndrome
— Fetal parvovirus syndrome
— Fetal phenothiazine syndrome
— Fetal prostaglandin syndrome
— Fetal thalidomide syndrome
— Fetal warfarin syndrome
— FG syndrome
— Fiber type disproportion, congenital
— Fibrinogen deficiency, congenital
— Fibrochondrogenesis
— Fibrolipomatosis
— Fibroma
— Fibromatosis gingival hypertrichosis
— Fibromatosis multiple non ossifying
— Fibromatosis
— Fibromuscular dysplasia of arteries
— Fibromuscular dysplasia
— Fibrosarcoma
— Fibrosing alveolitis
— Fibrosing Mediastinitis
— Fibrosis
— Fibrous dysplasia of bone
— Fibrous dysplasia
— Fibrodysplasia ossificans progressiva

— Fibula aplasia complex brachydactyly
— Fibular aplasia ectrodactyly
— Fibular hypoplasia femoral bowing oligodactyly
— Fibular hypoplasia scapulo pelvic dysplasia absent
— Filariasis
— Filippi syndrome
— Fine Lubinsky syndrome
— Fingerprints absence syndactyly milia
— Finnish lethal neonatal metabolic syndrome
— Finnish type amyloidosis
— Finucane Kurtz Scott syndrome
— Fish poisoning
— Fish-eye disease
— Fissured tongue
— Fistulous vegetative verrucous hydradenoma
— Fitz-Hugh-Curtis syndrome
— Fitzsimmons Walson Mellor syndrome
— Fitzsimmons-Guilbert syndrome
— Fitzsimmons-McLachlan-Gilbert syndrome
— Flavimonas oryzihabitans
— Flesh eating bacteria
— Floating limb syndrome
— Floating-harbor syndrome
— Florid cystic endosalpingiosis of the uterus
— Flotch syndrome
— Fluorosis
— Flynn Aird syndrome
— Focal agyria pachygyria
— Focal alopecia congenital megalencephaly
— Focal dermal hypoplasia
— Focal dystonia
— Focal facial dermal dysplasia
— Focal or multifocal malformations in neuronal migration
— Foix-Chavany-Marie syndrome
— Foix-Alajouanine syndrome
— Follicular atrophoderma-basal cell carcinoma
— Follicular Dendritic Cell Tumor
— Follicular hamartoma alopecia cystic fibrosis
— Follicular ichthyosis
— Follicular lymphoma

— Follicular lymphoreticuloma
— Fontaine Farriaux Blanckaert syndrome
— Forbes Albright syndrome
— Forbes disease
— Forestier's disease
— Formaldehyde poisoning
— Forney Robinson Pascoe syndrome
— Fountain syndrome
— Fowler Christmas Chapele syndrome
— Fox-Fordyce disease
— Fragile X syndrome type 1
— Fragile X syndrome type 2
— Fragile X syndrome type 3
— Fragile X syndrome
— Fragoso Cid Garcia Hernandez syndrome
— Franceschetti-Klein syndrome
— Francheschini Vardeu Guala syndrome
— Francois dyscephalic syndrome
— Franek Bocker kahlen syndrome
— Fraser Jequier Chen syndrome
— Fraser like syndrome
— Fraser syndrome
— Frasier syndrome
— FRAXA syndrome
— FRAXD
— FRAXE syndrome
— Free sialic acid storage disease
— Freeman-Sheldon syndrome
— Freiberg's disease
— Freire Maia odontotrichomelic syndrome
— Freire Maia Pinheiro Opitz syndrome
— Frenkel Russe syndrome
— Frey's syndrome
— Frias syndrome
— Fried Goldberg Mundel syndrome
— Friedel Heid Grosshans syndrome
— Friedman Goodman syndrome
— Friedreich ataxia congenital glaucoma
— Friedreich's ataxia
— Frigophobia

— Froelich's syndrome
— Frölich's syndrome
— Fronto nasal malformation cloacal exstrophy
— Frontofacionasal dysplasia type Al gazali
— Fronto-facio-nasal dysplasia
— Frontometaphyseal dysplasia
— Frontonasal dysplasia acromelic
— Frontonasal dysplasia klippel feil syndrome
— Frontonasal dysplasia phocomelic upper limbs
— Frontonasal dysplasia
— Frontotemporal dementia
— Fructosemia, hereditary
— fructosuria
— Frydman Cohen Ashenazi syndrome
— Frydman Cohen Karmon syndrome
— Fryer syndrome
— Fryns Fabry Remans syndrome
— Fryns Hofkens Fabry syndrome
— Fryns smeets thiry syndrome
— Fucosidosis type 1
— Fucosidosis
— Fuhrmann Rieger De sousa syndrome
— Fukuda Miyanomae Nakata syndrome
— Fukuyama type muscular dystrophy
— Fumarase deficiency
— Fumaric aciduria
— Functioning pancreatic endocrine tumor
— Fuqua Berkovitz syndrome
— Furlong Kurczynski Hennessy syndrome
— Furukawa Takagi Nakao syndrome
— Furunculous myiasis
— Fused mandibular incisors

G

— G syndrome
— Galactorrhea
— Galactocoele
— Galactokinase deficiency
— Galactorrhoea-Hyperprolactinaemia
— Galactosamine-6-sulfatase deficiency

— Galactose-1-phosphate uridyltransferase deficiency
— Galactosemia
— Galloway Mowat syndrome
— Gamborg Nielsen syndrome
— Game Friedman Paradice syndrome
— Gamma aminobutyric acid transaminase deficiency
— Gamma-cystathionase deficiency
— Gamma-sarcoglycanopathy
— Gamstorp episodic adynamy
— Ganglioglioma
— Gangliosidosis (Type2)(GM2)
— Gangliosidosis GM1 type 3
— Gangliosidosis type1
— GAPO syndrome
— Garcia Torres Guarner syndrome
— Gardner Morrisson Abbot syndrome
— Gardner Silengo Wachtel syndrome
— Gardner-Diamond syndrome
— Gardner's syndrome
— Garret Tripp syndrome
— Gas/bloat syndrome
— Gastric Dumping Syndrome
— Gastric lymphoma
— Gastritis, familial giant hypertrophic
— Gastrocutaneous syndrome
— Gastroenteritis, eosinophilic
— Gastro-enteropancreatic neuroendocrine tumor
— Gastroesophageal reflux
— Gastrointestinal autonomic nerve tumor
— Gastrointestinal neoplasm
— Gaucher disease type 1
— Gaucher disease type 2
— Gaucher disease type 3
— Gaucher Disease
— Gaucher ichthyosis restrictive dermopathy
— Gaucher-like disease
— Gaucher's disease
— Gay Feinmesser Cohen syndrome
— Geen Sandford Davison syndrome
— Gelatinous ascites

— Geleophysic dwarfism
— Gelineau disease
— Geliphobia
— Gemignani syndrome
— Gemss syndrome
— Genée-Wiedemann syndrome
— Generalized malformations in neuronal migration
— Generalized resistance to thyroid hormone
— Generalized seizure
— Generalized torsion dystonia
— Genes syndrome
— Genetic Diseases, Inborn
— Genetic reflex epilepsy
— Genetic susceptibility to infections caused by BCG
— Geniophobia
— Genital anomaly cardiomyopathy
— Genital dwarfism, Turner type
— Genital dwarfism
— Genito palatocardiac syndrome
— Genu valgum, st. Helena familial
— Genu varum
— Genuphobia
— Geographic tongue
— German syndrome
— Germinal cell aplasia
— Gerodermia osteodysplastica
— Gershinibaruch Leibo syndrome
— Gerstmann syndrome
— Gestational diabetes mellitus
— Gestational pemphigoid
— Gestational trophoblastic disease
— Ghosal syndrome
— Ghose Sachdev Kumar syndrome
— Gianotti-Crosti syndrome
— Giant axonal neuropathy
— Giant cell arteritis
— Giant cell myocarditis
— Giant congenital nevi
— Giant ganglionic hyperplasia
— Giant hypertrophic gastritis

— Giant mammary hamartoma
— Giant papillary conjunctivitis
— Giant pigmented hairy nevus
— Giant platelet syndrome
— Giardiasis
— Giedion syndrome
— Gigantism advanced bone age hoarse cry
— Gigantism partial, nevi, hemihypertrophy, macrocephaly
— Gigantism
— Gilbert's syndrome
— Gilles de la Tourette's syndrome
— Gingival fibromatosis dominant
— Gingival fibromatosis facial dysmorphism
— Gingival fibrosis
— Gingivitis
— Girate atrophy of choroid and retina
— Gitelman syndrome
— Glanzmann thrombasthenia
— Glass Chapman Hockley syndrome
— Glaucoma ecopia microspherophakia stiff joints short stature
— Glaucoma iridogoniodysgenesia
— Glaucoma sleep apnea
— Glaucoma type 1C
— Glaucoma, congenital
— Glaucoma, hereditary adult type 1A
— Glaucoma, hereditary juvenile type 1B
— Glaucoma, hereditary
— Glaucoma, primary infantile type 3A
— Glaucoma, primary infantile type 3B
— Glioblastoma multiforme
— Glioblastoma
— Glioma
— Gliomatosis cerebri
— Gliosarcoma
— Globel disaccharide intolerance
— Glomerulonephritis sparse hair telangiectases
— Glomerulonephritis
— Glomerulosclerosis
— Gloomy face syndrome
— Glossodynia

— Glossopalatine ankylosis micrognathia ear anomalies
— Glossopharyngeal neuralgia
— Glossophobia
— Glucagonoma
— Glucocorticoid deficiency, familial
— Glucocorticoid resistance
— Glucocorticoid sensitive hypertension
— Glucose 6 phosphate dehydrogenase deficiency
— Glucose-6-phosphate translocase deficiency
— Glucose-galactose malabsorption
— Glucosephosphate isomerase deficiency
— Glucosidase acid-1,4-alpha deficiency
— Glut2 deficiency
— Glutamate decarboxylase deficiency
— Glutamate-aspartate transport defect
— Glutaricaciduria I
— Glutaricaciduria II
— Glutaryl-CoA dehydrogenase deficiency
— Glyceraldehyde-3-phosphate dehydrogenase deficiency
— Glycine synthase deficiency
— Glycogen storage disease
— Glycogen storage disease type 1B
— Glycogen storage disease type 1C
— Glycogen storage disease type 1D
— Glycogen storage disease type 6, due to phosphorylation
— Glycogen storage disease type 7
— Glycogen storage disease type 9
— Glycogen storage disease type II
— Glycogen storage disease type V
— Glycogen storage disease type VI
— Glycogen storage disease type VII
— Glycogen storage disease type VIII
— Glycogenosis type II
— Glycogenosis type III
— Glycogenosis type IV
— Glycogenosis type V
— Glycogenosis type VI
— Glycogenosis type VII
— Glycogenosis type VIII
— Glycogenosis, type 0

— Glycosuria
— GM2 gangliosidosis, 0 variant
— GM2-gangliosidosis, B, B1, AB variant
— Gms syndrome
— Goiter
— Goldberg Bull syndrome
— Goldberg syndrome
— Goldblatt Wallis syndrome
— Goldblatt Wallis Zieff syndrome
— Goldblatt Viljoen syndrome
— Goldenhar syndrome
— Goldskag Cooks Hertz syndrome
— Goldstein Hutt syndrome
— Gollop Coates syndrome
— Gollop syndrome
— Goltz syndrome
— Gombo syndrome
— Gomez and López-Hernández syndrome
— Gonadal dysgenesis mixed
— Gonadal dysgenesis Turner type
— Gonadal dysgenesis XY type associated anomalies
— Gonadal dysgenesis, XX type
— Gonadal dysgenesis, XY female type
— Gonadal dysgenesis
— Goniodysgenesis mental retardation short stature
— Gonococcal conjunctivitis
— Gonzales Del Angel syndrome
— Goodman camptodactyly
— Goodpasture pneumorenal syndrome
— Goodpasture's syndrome
— Gordon hyperkaliemia-hypertension syndrome
— Gordon syndrome
— Gorham syndrome
— Gorham's disease
— Gorham-Stout disease
— Gorlin Bushkell Jensen syndrome
— Gorlin Chaudhry Moss syndrome
— Gottron's syndrome
— Gougerot-Sjogren syndrome
— Gouty nephropathy, familial

— Graft versus host disease
— Graham Boyle Troxell syndrome
— Grand Kaine Fulling syndrome
— Grant syndrome
— Granulocytopenia
— Granuloma annulare
— Granulomas, congenital cerebral
— Granulomatosis, lymphomatoid
— Granulomatous allergic angiitis
— Granulomatous hypophysitis
— Granulomatous rosacea
— Graphite Pneumoconiosis
— Graves' disease
— Gray platelet syndrome
— Great vessels transposition
— Greenberg dysplasia
— Greig cephalopolysyndactyly syndrome GCPS
— Griscelli disease
— Grix Blankenship Peterson syndrome
— Groll Hirschowitz syndrome
— Grosse syndrome
— Grover's disease
— Growth deficiency brachydactyly unusual facies
— Growth delay, constitutional
— Growth hormone deficiency
— Growth mental deficiency syndrome of Myhre
— Growth retardation alopecia pseudoanodontia optic
— Growth retardation hydrocephaly lung hypoplasia
— Growth retardation mental retardation phalangeal hypoplasia
— Grubben Decock Borghgraef syndrome
— GTP cyclohydrolase deficiency
— Guanidinoacetate methyltransferase deficiency
— Guérin-Stern syndrome
— Guibaud Vainsel syndrome
— Guillain-Barré syndrome
— Guizar Vasquez Luengas syndrome
— Guizar Vasquez Sanchez Manzano syndrome
— Gunal Seber Basaran syndrome
— Gupta Patton syndrome
— Gurrieri Sammito Bellussi syndrome

— Gusher syndrome
— Gymnophobia
— Gyrate atrophy of the retina
— Gyrate atrophy

H

— Hageman factor deficiency
— Hagemoser Weinstein Bresnick syndrome
— Hailey-Hailey disease
— Hair defect with photosensitivity and mental retardation
— Hairy cell leukemia
— Hairy ears, y-linked
— Hairy ears
— Hairy nose tip
— Hairy palms and soles
— Hairy tongue
— Hajdu-Cheney syndrome
— Halal Setton Wang syndrome
— Halal syndrome
— Hall Riggs mental retardation syndrome
— Hallermann Streiff syndrome
— Hallervorden-Spatz disease
— Hallux valgus
— Hamanishi Ueba Tsuji syndrome
— Hamano Tsukamoto syndrome
— Hamartoma sebaceus of Jadassohn
— Hand and foot deformity flat facies
— Hand foot uterus syndrome
— Hand wringing Rett syndrome
— Hand-foot-mouth disease
— Hand-Schuller-Christian disease
— Hanhart syndrome
— Hantavirosis
— Hantavirus pulmonary syndrome
— Hapnes Boman Skeie syndrome
— Hard skin syndrome Parana type
— HARD syndrome
— Harding ataxia
— Harlequin type ichthyosis
— Harpaxophobia

— Harrod Doman Keele syndrome
— Hartnup disease
— Hartsfield Bixler Demyer syndrome
— Hashimoto struma
— Hashimoto-Pritzker syndrome
— Hashimoto's thyroiditis
— Haspeslagh Fryns Muelenaere syndrome
— Hay Wells syndrome recessive type
— Hay-Wells syndrome
— Headache, cluster
— Hearing disorder
— Hearing impairment
— Hearing loss
— Heart aneurysm
— Heart block progressive, familial
— Heart block
— Heart defect round face congenital retarded development
— Heart defect tongue hamartoma polysyndactyly
— Heart defects limb shortening
— Heart hand syndrome Spanish type
— Heart hypertrophy, hereditary
— Heart situs anomaly
— Heart tumor of the adult
— Heart tumor of the child
— Heavy metal poisoning
— Hec syndrome
— Hecht Scott syndrome
— Heckenlively syndrome
— Heide syndrome
— Heliophobia
— HELLP syndrome
— Helmerhorst Heaton Crossen syndrome
— Helminthiasis
— HEM dysplasia
— Hemangioblastoma
— Hemangioendothelioma
— Hemangioma thrombocytopenia syndrome
— Hemangioma, capillary infantile
— Hemangioma
— Hemangiomatosis, familial pulmonary capillary

- Hemangiopericytoma
- Hemeralopia, congenital essential
- Hemeralopia, familial
- Hemi 3 syndrome
- Hemifacial atrophy agenesis of the caudate nucleus
- Hemifacial atrophy progressive
- Hemifacial hyperplasia strabismus
- Hemifacial microsomia
- Hemihypertrophy in context of NF
- Hemihypertrophy intestinal web corneal opacity
- Hemimegalencephaly
- Hemiplegia
- Hemiplegic migraine, familial
- Hemoglobin C disease
- Hemoglobin E disease
- Hemoglobin SC disease
- Hemoglobinopathy
- Hemoglobinuria
- Hemolytic anemia lethal genital anomalies
- Hemolytic-uremic syndrome
- Hemophagocytic lymphohistiocytosis
- Hemophagocytic reticulosis
- Hemophilia A
- Hemophilic arthropathy
- Hemophobia
- Hemorragic fever with renal syndrome
- Hemorrhagic fever
- Hemorrhagic proctocolitis
- Hemorrhagic thrombocythemia
- Hemorrhagiparous thrombocytic dystrophy
- Hemosiderosis
- Hemothorax
- Hennekam Beemer syndrome
- Hennekam Koss de Geest syndrome
- Hennekam syndrome
- Hennekam Van der Horst syndrome
- Hepadnovirus D
- Heparane sulfamidase deficiency
- Heparin-induced thrombopenia
- Hepatic cystic hamartoma

— Hepatic ductular hypoplasia
— Hepatic encephalopathy
— Hepatic fibrosis renal cysts mental retardation
— Hepatic fibrosis
— Hepatic venoocclusive disease
— Hepatic veno-occlusive disease
— Hepatitis A
— Hepatitis B
— Hepatitis C
— Hepatitis D
— Hepatitis non-A non-B
— Hepatitis non-A
— Hepatitis non-B
— Hepatitis, chronic autoimmune
— Hepatitis
— Hepatoblastoma
— Hepatocellular carcinoma
— Hepatorenal syndrome
— Hepatorenal tyrosinemia
— Hereditary amyloidosis
— Hereditary angioedema
— Hereditary ataxia
— Hereditary carnitine deficiency myopathy
— Hereditary carnitine deficiency syndrome
— Hereditary carnitine deficiency
— Hereditary ceroid lipofuscinosis
— Hereditary coproporphyria
— Hereditary deafness
— Hereditary elliptocytosis
— Hereditary fructose intolerance
— Hereditary hearing disorder
— Hereditary hearing loss
— Hereditary hemochromatosis
— Hereditary hemorrhagic telangiectasia
— Hereditary hyperuricemia
— Hereditary macrothrombocytopenia
— Hereditary methemoglobinemia, recessive
— Hereditary nodular heterotopia
— Hereditary non-spherocytic hemolytic anemia
— Hereditary pancreatitis

— Hereditary paroxysmal cerebral ataxia
— Hereditary peripheral nervous disorder
— Hereditary primary Fanconi disease
— Hereditary resistance to anti-vitamin K
— Hereditary sensory and autonomic neuropathy 3
— Hereditary sensory and autonomic neuropathy 4
— Hereditary sensory neuropathy type I
— Hereditary sensory neuropathy type II
— Hereditary spastic paraplegia
— Hereditary spherocytic hemolytic anemia
— Hereditary spherocytosis
— Hereditary type 1 neuropathy
— Hereditary type 2 neuropathy
— Hermansky-Pudlak syndrome
— Hermaphroditism
— Hernandez Aguire Negrete syndrome
— Herpangina
— Herpes encephalitis
— Herpes simplex disease
— Herpes simplex encephalitis
— Herpes viridae disease
— Herpes virus antenatal infection
— Herpes zoster oticus
— Herpes zoster
— Herpesvirus simiae B virus
— Herpetic embryopathy
— Herpetic keratitis
— Herpetophobia
— Herrmann Opitz arthrogryposis syndrome
— Herrmann Opitz craniosynostosis
— Hers disease
— Hersh Podruch Weisskopk syndrome
— Heterophobia
— Heterotaxia (generic term)
— Heterotaxia autosomal dominant type
— Heterotaxy with polysplenia or asplenia
— Heterotaxy, visceral, X-linked
— Hexosaminidases A and B deficiency
— HHH syndrome
— Hibernian fever, familial

— Hiccups
— Hidradenitis suppurativa familial
— Hidradenitis suppurativa
— Hidrotic ectodermal dysplasia type Christianson Fouris
— High scapula
— High-molecular-weight kininogen deficiency, congenital
— Hillig syndrome
— Hing Torack Dowston syndrome
— Hinson-Pepys disease
— Hip dislocation
— Hip dysplasia Beukes type
— Hip dysplasia
— Hip luxation
— Hip subluxation
— Hipo syndrome
— Hirschsprung disease ganglioneuroblastoma
— Hirschsprung disease polydactyly heart disease
— Hirschsprung disease type 2
— Hirschsprung disease type 3
— Hirschsprung disease type d brachydactyly
— Hirschsprung microcephaly cleft palate
— Hirschsprung nail hypoplasia dysmorphism
— Hirschsprung's disease
— Hirsutism congenital gingival hyperplasia
— Hirsutism skeletal dysplasia mental retardation
— His bundle tachycardia
— Histidinemia
— Histidinuria renal tubular defect
— Histiocytosis X
— Histiocytosis, Non-Langerhans-Cell
— Histoplasmosis
— Hittner Hirsch Kreh syndrome
— Hm syndrome
— HMG CoA lyase deficiency
— HMG CoA synthetase deficiency
— Hodgkin lymphoma
— Hodgkin's disease
— Hodophobia
— Hoepffner Dreyer Reimers syndrome
— Hollow visceral myopathy

— Holmes Benacerraf syndrome
— Holmes Borden syndrome
— Holmes Collins syndrome
— Holmes Gang syndrome
— Holoacardius amorphus
— Holocarboxylase synthetase deficiency
— Holoprosencephaly caudal dysgenesis
— Holoprosencephaly deletion 2p
— Holoprosencephaly ectrodactyly cleft lip palate
— Holoprosencephaly radial heart renal anomalies
— Holoprosencephaly
— Holt-Oram syndrome
— Holzgreve Wagner Rehder syndrome
— Homocarnosinase deficiency
— Homocarnosinosis
— Homocystinuria due to cystathionine beta-synthase
— Homocystinuria due to defect in methylation (cbl g)
— Homocystinuria due to defect in methylation cbl e
— Homocystinuria due to defect in methylation, MTHFR deficiency
— Homocystinuria
— Homologous wasting disease
— Homozygous hypobetalipoproteinemia
— Hoon Hall syndrome
— Hordnes Engebretsen Knudtson syndrome
— Horn Kolb syndrome
— Horner's syndrome
— Hornova Dlurosova syndrome
— Horseshoe kidney
— Horton disease, juvenile
— Horton disease
— Houlston Ironton Temple syndrome
— Howard Young syndrome
— Howell-Evans syndrome
— Hoyeraal Hreidarsson syndrome
— Hoyeraal syndrome
— HSV-2 infection
— Human granulocytic ehrlichiosis
— Human monocytic ehrlichiosis
— Human parvovirus B19 infection
— Humero spinal dysostosis congenital heart disease

— Humeroradial synostosis
— Humeroradioulnar synostosis
— Humerus trochlea aplasia of
— Hunter Carpenter Mc donald syndrome
— Hunter Jurenka Thompson syndrome
— Hunter Macpherson syndrome
— Hunter Mcalpine syndrome
— Hunter Mcdonald syndrome
— Hunter Rudd Hoffmann syndrome
— Hunter syndrome
— Huntington's disease
— Huriez scleroatrophic syndrome
— Hurler syndrome
— Hurst Hallam Hockey syndrome
— Hutchinson Gilford Progeria Syndrome
— Hutchinson incisors
— Hutchinson-Gilford syndrome
— Hutteroth Spranger syndrome
— Hyalinosis systemic short stature
— Hyaloideoretinal degeneration of wagner
— Hydantoin antenatal infection
— Hydatidiform mole
— Hydatidosis
— Hyde Forster Mccarthy Berry syndrome
— Hydranencephaly
— Hydrocephalus - Arnold Chiari - allied disorders
— Hydrocephalus autosomal recessive
— Hydrocephalus costovertebral dysplasia Sprengel anomaly
— Hydrocephalus craniosynostosis bifid nose
— Hydrocephalus endocardial fibroelastosis cataract
— Hydrocephalus growth retardation skeletal anomalies
— Hydrocephalus obesity hypogonadism
— Hydrocephalus skeletal anomalies
— Hydrocephalus
— Hydrocephaly corpus callosum agenesis diaphragmatic hernia
— Hydrocephaly low insertion umbilicus
— Hydrocephaly tall stature joint laxity
— Hydrolethalus syndrome
— Hydronephrosis
— Hydronephrosis peculiar facial expression

— Hydrophobia
— Hydrops ectrodactyly syndactyly
— Hydrops fetalis anemia immune disorder absent thumb
— Hydrops fetalis
— Hydroxycarboxylic aciduria
— Hydroxymethylglutaricaciduria
— Hygroma cervical
— Hymenolepiasis
— Hyper IgE
— Hyper IgM syndrome
— Hyperadrenalism
— Hyperaldosteronism familial type 2
— Hyperaldosteronism, familial type 1
— Hyperaldosteronism
— Hyperammonemia
— Hyperandrogenism
— Hyperbilirubinemia transient familial neonatal
— Hyperbilirubinemia type 1
— Hyperbilirubinemia type 2
— Hyperbilirubinemia
— Hypercalcemia, familial benign type 1
— Hypercalcemia, familial benign type 2
— Hypercalcemia, familial benign type 3
— Hypercalcemia, familial benign
— Hypercalcemia
— Hypercalcinuria idiopathic
— Hypercalcinuria macular coloboma
— Hypercalcinuria
— Hypercementosis
— Hypercholesterolemia due to arg3500 mutation of Apo B-100
— Hypercholesterolemia due to LDL receptor deficiency
— Hypercholesterolemia
— Hyperchylomicronemia
— Hypereosinophilic syndrome
— Hyperexplexia
— Hyperferritinemia, hereditary, with congenital cataracts
— Hypergeusia
— Hyperglycemia
— Hyperglycerolemia
— Hyperglycinemia, isolated nonketotic type 1

— Hyperglycinemia, isolated nonketotic type 2
— Hyperglycinemia, isolated nonketotic
— Hyperglycinemia
— Hypergonadotropic ovarian failure, familial or sporadic
— Hyperhidrosis
— Hyperhomocysteinemia
— Hyper-IgD syndrome
— Hyperimidodipeptiduria
— Hyperimmunoglobinemia D with recurrent fever
— Hyperimmunoglobulin E - reccurrent infection syndrome
— Hyperimmunoglobulinemia D with periodic fever
— Hyperimmunoglobulinemia E
— Hyperinsulinism due to focal adenomatous hyperplasia
— Hyperinsulinism due to glucokinase deficiency
— Hyperinsulinism due to glutamodehydrogenase deficiency
— Hyperinsulinism in children, congenital
— Hyperinsulinism, diffuse
— Hyperinsulinism, focal
— Hyperkalemia
— Hyperkalemic periodic paralysis
— Hyperkeratosis lenticularis perstans of Flegel
— Hyperkeratosis lenticularis perstans
— Hyperkeratosis palmoplantar localized acanthokeratolytic
— Hyperkeratosis palmoplantar localized epidermolytic
— Hyperkeratosis palmoplantar with palmar crease hyperkeratosis
— Hyperlipoproteinemia type I
— Hyperlipoproteinemia type II
— Hyperlipoproteinemia type III
— Hyperlipoproteinemia type IV
— Hyperlipoproteinemia type V
— Hyperlipoproteinemia
— Hyperlysinemia
— Hyperornithinemia
— Hyperornithinemia-hyperammonemia-homocitrullinuria
— Hyperostosid corticalis deformans juvenilis
— Hyperostosis cortical infantile
— Hyperostosis corticalis generalisata
— Hyperostosis frontalis interna
— Hyperoxaluria type 1
— Hyperoxaluria type 2

— Hyperoxaluria
— Hyperparathyroidism, familial, primary
— Hyperparathyroidism, neonatal severe primary
— Hyperparathyroidism
— Hyperphalangism dysmorphy bronchomalacia
— Hyperphenilalaninemia due to pterin-4-alpha-carbin
— Hyperphenylalalinemia due to dihydropteridine reductase deficiency
— Hyperphenylalaninemia due to 6-pyruvoyltetrahydrop
— Hyperphenylalaninemia due to dehydratase deficiency
— Hyperphenylalaninemia due to GTP cyclohydrolase deficiency
— Hyperphenylalaninemic embryopathy
— Hyperpipecolatemia
— Hyperprolactinemia
— Hyperprolinemia type II
— Hyperprolinemia
— Hyperreflexia
— Hyper-reninism
— Hypersomnolence
— Hypertelorism and tetralogy of Fallot
— Hypertrichosis atrophic skin ectropion macrostomia
— Hypertropia
— Hypertropic neuropathy of Dejerine-Sottas
— Hypertryptophanemia
— Hypoadrenalism
— Hypoadrenocorticism hypoparathyroidism moniliasis
— Hypoaldosteronism
— Hypo-alphalipoproteinemia primary
— Hypobetalipoproteinaemia ataxia hearing loss
— Hypobetalipoprotéinemia, familial
— Hypocalcemia, autosomal dominant
— Hypocalcemia
— Hypocalcinuric hypercalcemia, familial
— Hypochondrogenesis
— Hypochondroplasia
— Hypocomplementemic urticarial vasculitis
— Hypodermyasis
— Hypodontia dysplasia of nails
— Hypodontia of incisors and premolars
— Hypofibrinogenemia, familial

— Hypoglycemia with deficiency of glycogen synthetase in the liver
— Hypoglycemia
— Hypogonadism cardiomyopathy
— Hypogonadism hypogonadotropic due to mutations in GR hormone
— Hypogonadism male mental retardation skeletal anomaly
— Hypogonadism mitral valve prolapse mental retardation
— Hypogonadism primary partial alopecia
— Hypogonadism retinitis pigmentosa
— Hypogonadism, isolated, hypogonadotropic
— Hypogonadism
— Hypogonadotropic hypogonadism syndactyly
— Hypogonadotropic hypogonadism without anosmia, X linked
— Hypogonadotropic hypogonadism-anosmia, X linked
— Hypogonadotropic hypogonadism-anosmia
— Hypohidrotic Ectodermal Dysplasia
— Hypokalemia
— Hypokalemic alkalosis with hypercalcinuria
— Hypokalemic periodic paralysis
— Hypokaliemic periodic paralysis type 1
— Hypoketonemic hypoglycemia
— Hypolipoproteinemia
— Hypomagnesemia primary
— Hypomandibular faciocranial dysostosis
— Hypomelanotic disorder
— Hypomelia mullerian duct anomalies
— Hypomentia
— Hypoparathyroidism familial isolated
— Hypoparathyroidism nerve deafness nephrosis
— Hypoparathyroidism short stature mental retardation
— Hypoparathyroidism short stature
— Hypoparathyroidism X linked
— Hypoparathyroidism
— Hypophosphatasia, infantile
— Hypophosphatasia
— Hypophosphatemic rickets
— Hypopigmentation oculocerebral syndrome Cross type
— Hypopituitarism micropenis cleft lip palate
— Hypopituitarism postaxial polydactyly

— Hypopituitarism
— Hypopituitary dwarfism
— Hypoplasia hepatic ductular
— Hypoplasia of the tibia with polydactyly
— Hypoplastic left heart syndrome
— Hypoplastic right heart microcephaly
— Hypoplastic thumb mullerian aplasia
— Hypoplastic thumbs hydranencephaly
— Hypoproconvertinemia
— Hypoprothrombinemia
— Hyporeninemic hypoaldosteronism
— Hyposmia nasal hypoplasia hypogonadism
— Hypospadias familial
— Hypospadias mental retardation Goldblatt type
— Hypotelorism cleft palate hypospadias
— Hypothalamic dysfunction
— Hypothalamic hamartoblastoma syndrome
— Hypothalamic hamartomas
— Hypothermia
— Hypothyroidism due to iodide transport defect
— Hypothyroidism postaxial polydactyly mental retardation
— Hypothyroidism
— Hypotonic sclerotic muscular dystrophy
— Hypotrichosis mental retardation Lopes type
— Hypotrichosis
— Hypotropia
— Hypoxanthine guanine phosphoribosyltransferase deficiency
— Hypoxia

I

— IBIDS syndrome
— ICF syndrome
— Ichthyophobia
— Ichthyosiform erythroderma corneal involvement deafness
— Ichthyosis alopecia eclabion ectropion mental retardation
— Ichthyosis and male hypogonadism
— Ichthyosis bullosa of Siemens
— Ichthyosis cheek eyebrow syndrome
— Ichthyosis congenita biliary atresia
— Ichthyosis deafness mental retardation skeletal anomaly

— Ichthyosis follicularis atrichia photophobia syndrome
— Ichthyosis hepatosplenomegaly cerebellar degeneration
— Ichthyosis hystrix, Curth Macklin type
— Ichthyosis linearis circumflexa
— Ichthyosis male hypogonadism
— Ichthyosis mental retardation Devriendt type
— Ichthyosis mental retardation dwarfism renal impairment
— Ichthyosis microphthalmos
— Ichthyosis tapered fingers midline groove up
— Ichthyosis vulgaris
— Ichthyosis, erythrokeratolysis hemalis
— Ichthyosis, keratosis follicularis spinulosa Decalvans
— Ichthyosis, lamellar recessive
— Ichthyosis, Netherton syndrome
— Idaho syndrome
— Idiopathic acute eosinophilic pneumonia
— Idiopathic adolescent scoliosis
— Idiopathic adult neutropenia
— Idiopathic alveolar hypoventilation syndrome
— Idiopathic congenital nystagmus, dominant, X- linked
— Idiopathic diffuse interstitial fibrosis
— Idiopathic dilatation of the pulmonary artery
— Idiopathic dilation cardiomyopathy
— Idiopathic double athetosis
— Idiopathic edema
— Idiopathic eosinophilic chronic pneumopathy
— Idiopathic facial palsy
— Idiopathic hypereosinophilic syndrome
— Idiopathic infection caused by BCG or atypical mycobacteria
— Idiopathic juvenile osteoporosis
— Idiopathic pulmonary fibrosis
— Idiopathic pulmonary hemosiderosis
— Idiopathic sclerosing mesenteritis
— Idiopathic thrombocytopenic purpura
— Iduronate 2-sulfatase deficiency
— IFAP syndrome
— IgA deficiency
— IGDA syndrome
— Illum syndrome
— Illyngophobia

— Ilyina Amoashy Grygory syndrome
— Imaizumi Kuroki syndrome
— Iminoglycinuria
— Immotile cilia syndrome, due to defective radial spokes
— Immotile cilia syndrome, due to excessively long cilia
— Immotile cilia syndrome, Kartagener type
— Immune deficiency, familial variable
— Immune thrombocytopenia
— Immunodeficiency, primary
— Immunodeficiency, secondary
— Immunodeficiency with short limb dwarfism
— Immunodeficiency, microcephaly with normal intelligence
— Imperforate anus
— Imperforate oropharynx costo vetebral anomalies
— Impossible syndrome
— Inactive colon
— Inborn amino acid metabolism disorder
— Inborn branched chain aminoaciduria
— Inborn error of metabolism
— Inborn metabolic disorder
— Inborn renal aminoaciduria
— Inborn urea cycle disorder
— Incisors fused
— Inclusion conjunctivitis
— Incontinentia pigmenti type 1
— Incontinentia pigmenti type 2
— Incontinentia pigmenti
— Indomethacin antenatal infection
— Infant epilepsy with migrant focal crisis
— Infant respiratory distress syndrome
— Infantile apnea
— Infantile axonal neuropathy
— Infantile convulsions and paroxysmal choreoathetosis, familial
— Infantile digital fibromatosis
— Infantile dysphagia
— Infantile multisystem inflammatory disease
— Infantile myofibromatosis
— Infantile onset spinocerebellar ataxia
— Infantile recurrent chronic multifocal osteomyolitis
— Infantile sialic acid storage disorder

— Infantile spasms broad thumbs
— Infantile spasms
— Infantile spinal muscular atrophy
— Infantile striato thalamic degeneration
— Infectious arthritis
— Infectious myocarditis
— Infective endocarditis
— Inflammatory breast cancer
— Infundibulopelvic stenosis multicystic kidney
— Influenza
— Inguinal hernia
— Insensitivity to pain with anhidrosis
— Instability mitotic non disjunction syndrome
— Insulinoma
— Insulin-resistance type B
— Insulin-resistant acanthosis nigricans, type A
— Intercellular cholesterol esterification disease
— Interferon gamma, receptor 1, deficiency
— Internal carotid agenesis
— Interstitial cystitis
— Interstitial pneumonia
— Intestinal atresia multiple
— Intestinal lipodystrophy
— Intestinal lymphangiectasia
— Intestinal malrotation facial anomalies familial type
— Intestinal pseudoobstruction chronic idiopathic
— Intestinal pseudo-obstruction
— Intoeing
— Intracranial aneurysms multiple congenital anomaly
— Intracranial arterioveinous malformation
— Intractable singultus
— Intrathoracic kidney vertebral fusion
— Intrauterine growth retardation mandibular malar hypoplasia
— Intrauterine infections
— Intrinsic factor, congenital deficiency of
— Iodine antenatal infection
— Iodine deficiency
— Iophobia
— Iridocyclitis
— Iridogoniodysgenesis, dominant type

— Iris dysplasia hypertelorism deafness
— Iritis
— Irons Bhan syndrome
— Irritable bowel syndrome
— Isaacs Mertens syndrome
— Isaacs syndrome
— Ischiadic hypoplasia renal dysfunction immunodeficiency
— Ischiopatellar dysplasia
— Isosporosiasis
— Isotretinoin embryopathy
— Isthmian coarctation
— Ivemark syndrome
— Ivic Syndrome

J

— Jackson-Weiss syndrome
— Jacobsen syndrome
— Jadassohn Lewandowsky syndrome
— Jaffer Beighton syndrome
— Jalili syndrome
— Jancar syndrome
— Jankovic Rivera syndrome
— Jansen type metaphyseal chondrodysplasia
— Jansky-Bielschowsky disease
— Japanese encephalitis
— Jarcho-Levin syndrome
— Jejunal atresia
— Jensen syndrome
— Jequier Kozlowski skeletal dysplasia
— Jervell Lange-Nielsen syndrome
— Jeune syndrome situs inversus
— Jeune syndrome
— Job syndrome
— Johanson Blizzard syndrome
— Johnson Hall Krous syndrome
— Johnson Munson syndrome
— Johnston Aarons Schelley syndrome
— Jones Hersh Yusk syndrome
— Jones syndrome
— Jorgenson Lenz syndrome

— Joseph disease
— Joubert syndrome bilateral chorioretinal coloboma
— Joubert syndrome
— Juberg Hayward syndrome
— Juberg Marsidi syndrome
— Judge Misch Wright syndrome
— Jumping Frenchmen of Maine
— Jung Wolff Back Stahl syndrome
— Juvenile cataract cerebellar atrophy myopathy mental retardation
— Juvenile dermatomyositis
— Juvenile gastrointestinal polyposis
— Juvenile gout
— Juvenile hyaline fibromatosis
— Juvenile macular degeneration hypotrichosis
— Juvenile muscular atrophy of the distal upper limb
— Juvenile myoclonic epilepsy
— Juvenile nephronophthisis
— Juvenile rheumatoid arthritis
— Juvenile temporal arteritis

K

— Kabuki syndrome
— Kalam Hafeez syndrome
— Kaler Garrity Stern syndrome
— Kallikrein hypertension
— Kallmann syndrome with Spastic paraplegia
— Kallmann syndrome with heart disease
— Kallmann syndrome, type 1, X linked
— Kallmann syndrome, type 3, recessive
— Kalyanraman syndrome
— Kantaputra Gorlin syndrome
— Kaolin pneumoconiosis
— Kaplan Plauchu Fitch syndrome
— Kaplowitz Bodurtha syndrome
— Kaposi sarcoma
— Kaposiform hemangio-endothelioma
— Kapur Toriello syndrome
— Karandikar Maria Kamble syndrome
— Karsch Neugebauer syndrome

— Kartagener syndrome
— Kashani Strom Utley syndrome
— Kasznica Carlson Coppedge syndrome
— Kathisophobia
— Katsantoni Papadakou Lagoyanni syndrome
— Katz syndrome
— Kaufman oculocerebrofacial syndrome
— Kawasaki syndrome
— KBG syndrome
— Kearns-Sayre syndrome
— Keloids
— Kennedy disease
— Kennerknecht Sorgo Oberhoffer syndrome
— Kennerknecht Vogel syndrome
— Kenny Caffey syndrome
— Kenny-Caffey syndrome, Type 1
— Keratitis, hereditary
— Keratoacanthoma familial
— Keratoacanthoma
— Keratoconjunctivitis sicca
— Keratoconus posticus circumscriptus
— Keratoconus
— Keratoderma hypotrichosis leukonychia
— Keratoderma palmoplantar deafness
— Keratoderma palmoplantar spastic paralysis
— Keratoderma palmoplantaris transgrediens
— Keratolytic winter erythema
— Keratomalacia
— Keratosis focal palmoplantar gingival
— Keratosis follicularis dwarfism cerebral atrophy
— Keratosis follicularis spinulosa decalvans
— Keratosis palmoplantaris adenocarcinoma of the colon
— Keratosis palmoplantaris esophageal colon cancer
— Keratosis palmoplantaris papulosa
— Keratosis palmoplantaris with corneal dystrophy
— Keratosis palmoplantar-periodontopathy
— Keratosis pilaris
— Keratosis, seborrheic
— Kerion celsi
— Kernicterus

— Keutel syndrome
— Ki-1cell lymphoma
— KID syndrome
— Kifafa seizure disorder
— Kikuchi disease
— Kimura disease
— King-Denborough syndrome
— Kleeblattschaedel syndrome
— Kleine Levin Syndrome
— Kleiner Holmes syndrome
— Klinefelter's Syndrome
— Klippel Feil deformity conductive deafness absent vagina
— Klippel Feil syndrome dominant type
— Klippel Feil syndrome recessive type
— Klippel Trenaunay Weber syndrome
— Klippel-Feil syndrome
— Klumpke paralysis
— Klüver-Bucy syndrome
— Kniest dysplasia
— Kniest like dysplasia lethal
— Knobloch-Layer syndrome
— Knuckle pads, leuconychia and sensorineural deafness
— Kobberling-Dunnigan syndrome
— Kocher-Debré-Semélaigne syndrome
— Kohler disease
— Kohlschutter Tonz syndrome
— Konigsmark Knox Hussels syndrome
— Koone Rizzo Elias syndrome
— Korsakoff's syndrome
— Korula Wilson Salomonson syndrome
— Kostmann syndrome
— Kosztolanyi syndrome
— Kotzot-Richter syndrome
— Kousseff Nichols syndrome
— Kousseff syndrome
— Kowarski syndrome
— Kozlowski Brown Hardwick syndrome
— Kozlowski Celermajer syndrome
— Kozlowski Massen syndrome
— Kozlowski Ouvrier syndrome

— Kozlowski Rafinski Klicharska syndrome
— Kozlowski Tsuruta Taki syndrome
— Kozlowski Warren Fisher syndrome
— Kozlowski-Krajewska syndrome
— Krabbe leukodystrophy
— Krasnow Qazi syndrome
— Krause-Kivlin syndrome
— Krauss Herman Holmes syndrome
— Krieble Bixler syndrome
— Kumar Levick syndrome
— Kurczynski Casperson syndrome
— Kuskokwim disease
— Kuster Majewski Hammerstein syndrome
— Kuster syndrome
— Kuzniecky syndrome
— Kyasanur Forrest disease
— Kyphosis
— Kyphosis brachyphalangy optic atrophy

L

— Labrador lung
— Labyrinthitis
— Lachiewicz Sibley syndrome
— Lacrimo-auriculo-dento-digital syndrome
— Lactate dehydrogenase deficiency type A
— Lactate dehydrogenase deficiency type B
— Lactate dehydrogenase deficiency type C
— Lactate dehydrogenase deficiency
— Lactic acidosis congenital infantile
— Ladda Zonana Ramer syndrome
— Lafora disease
— Lagophthalmia cleft lip palate
— Lambdoid synostosis familial
— Lambert syndrome
— Lambert-Eaton Myasthenic Syndrome (Lambert-Eaton paraneoplastic cerebellar degeneration)
— Lambert-Eaton syndrome
— Lamellar ichthyosis
— Lamellar recessive ichthyosis
— Landau-Kleffner syndrome

— Landouzy-Dejerine muscular dystrophy
— Landy Donnai syndrome
— Langdon Down
— Langer Nishino Yamaguchi syndrome
— Langer-Giedion syndrome
— Langerhans cell granulomatosis
— Langerhans cell histiocytosis
— Laparoschisis
— Laplane Fontaine Lagardere syndrome
— Large B cell diffuse lymphoma
— Laron-type dwarfism
— Larsen like osseous dysplasia dwarfism
— Larsen like syndrome lethal type
— Larsen syndrome craniosynostosis
— Larsen syndrome, dominant type
— Larsen syndrome, recessive type
— Larsen syndrome
— Laryngeal abductor paralysis mental retardation
— Laryngeal carcinoma
— Laryngeal cleft
— Laryngeal neoplasm
— Laryngeal papillomatosis
— Laryngeal web congenital heart disease short stature
— Laryngocele
— Laryngomalacia dominant congenital
— Laryngomalacia
— Larynx atresia
— Lassa fever
— Lassueur-Graham-Little syndrome
— Late onset dominant cone dystrophy
— Lateral body wall defect
— Laterality defects dominant
— Lattice corneal dystrophy type 2
— Launois-Bensaude adenolipomatosis
— Laurence Prosser Rocker syndrome
— Laurence-Moon-Bardet-Biedl syndrome
— Laurin Sandrow syndrome
— Laxova Brown Hogan syndrome
— LBWC - amniotic bands
— LBWD syndrome

- LCHAD deficiency
- Leao Ribeiro Da Silva syndrome
- Learman syndrome
- Leber military aneurysm
- Leber optic atrophy
- Leber's Disease
- Lecithin cholesterol acyltransferase deficiency
- Ledderhose disease
- Lee Root Fenske syndrome
- Left ventricle-aorta tunnel
- Leg absence deformity cataract
- Legg-Calvé-Perthes syndrome
- Legionellosis
- Legionnaire's disease
- Lehman syndrome
- Leichtman Wood Rohn syndrome
- Leifer Lai Buyse syndrome
- Leigh disease
- Leigh syndrome, French Canadian type
- Leiner disease
- Leiomyoma
- Leiomyomatosis familial
- Leiomyomatosis of oesophagus cataract hematuria
- Leiomyosarcoma
- Leipala Kaitila syndrome
- Leishmaniasis
- Leisti Hollister Rimoin syndrome
- Lemierre's syndrome
- Lennox-Gastaut syndrome
- Lentiginosis in context of NF
- Lenz Majewski hyperostotic dwarfism
- Lenz microphthalmia syndrome
- Leprechaunism
- Leprosy
- Leptomeningeal capillary - venous angiomatosis
- Leptospirosis
- Leri pleonosteosis
- Leri-Weil syndrome
- Lesch-Nyhan syndrome
- Lethal chondrodysplasia Moerman type

— Lethal chondrodysplasia Seller type
— Lethal congenital contracture syndrome
— Letterer-Siwe disease
— Leucinosis
— Leukemia subleukemic
— Leukemia, B-Cell, chronic
— Leukemia, Myeloid
— Leukemia, T-Cell, chronic
— Leukemia
— Leukocyte adhesion deficiency syndrome
— Leukocyte adhesion deficiency type 2
— Leukocytoclastic angiitis
— Leukodystrophy reunion type
— Leukodystrophy, globoid cell
— Leukodystrophy, metachromatic
— Leukodystrophy, psuedometachromatic
— Leukodystrophy, Sudanophilic
— Leukodystrophy
— Leukoencephalopathy palmoplantar keratoderma
— Leukomalacia
— Leukomelanoderma mental retardation hypotrichosis
— Leukoplakia
— Levator syndrome
— Levic Stefanovic Nikolic syndrome
— Levine Crichley syndrome
— Lewandowski Kikolich syndrome
— Lewis Pashayan syndrome
— Leydig cells hypoplasia
— LGCR
— LGS
— Lhermitte-Duclos disease
— Lichen myxedematosus
— Lichen planus follicularis
— Lichen planus
— Lichen sclerosis et atrophicus
— Lichen spinulosus
— Lichstenstein syndrome
— Lida Kannari syndrome
— Liddle syndrome
— Li-Fraumeni syndrome

— Light chain disease
— Ligyrophobia
— Limb deficiencies distal micrognathia
— Limb dystonia
— Limb reduction defect
— Limb scalp and skull defects
— Limb transversal defect cardiac anomaly
— Limb-body wall complex
— Limb-girdle muscular dystrophy
— Limnophobia
— Lindsay Burn syndrome
— Lindstrom syndrome
— Linear hamartoma syndrome
— Linear nevus syndrome
— Linonophobia
— Lip lit syndrome
— Lipid storage myopathy
— Lipidosis with triglycerid storage disease
— Lipoamide dehydrogenase deficiency
— Lipodystrophy Rieger anomaly diabetes
— Lipodystrophy
— Lipogranulomatosis
— Lipoid congenital adrenal hyperplasia
— Lipoid proteinosis of Urbach and Wiethe
— Lipomatosis central non-encapsulated
— Lipomatosis familial benign cervical
— Lipomucopolysaccharidosis
— Lipoprotein disorder
— Liposarcoma
— Lisker Garcia Ramos syndrome
— Lison Kornbrut Feinstein syndrome
— Lissencephaly immunodeficiency
— Lissencephaly syndrome type 1
— Lissencephaly syndrome type 2
— Lissencephaly, isolated
— Lissencephaly
— Listeria infection
— Listeriosis
— Liticaphobia
— Liver cirrhosis

— Liver neoplasms
— Lobar atrophy of brain
— Lobster hand
— Lobstein disease
— Localized epiphyseal dysplasia
— Locked-In syndrome
— Lockwood Feingold syndrome
— Loffredo Cennamo Cecio syndrome
— Logic syndrome
— Loiasis
— Loin pain hematuria syndrome
— Long QT syndrome type 1
— Long QT syndrome type 2
— Long QT syndrome type 3
— Long QT Syndrome
— Loose anagen hair syndrome
— Loose anagene syndrome
— Lopes Gorlin syndrome
— Lopes Marques de Faria syndrome
— Lopez Hernandez syndrome
— Lou Gehrig's disease
— Louis Bar syndrome
— Low birth weight dwarfism dysgammaglobulinemia
— Lowe Kohn Cohen syndrome
— Lowe oculocerebrorenal syndrome
— Lowe syndrome
— Lower limb anomaly ureteral obstruction
— Lower limb deficiency hypospadias
— Lower mesodermal defects
— Lowry Maclean syndrome
— Lowry syndrome
— Lowry Wood syndrome
— Lowry Yong syndrome
— LSA
— L-transposition and ccTGA
— Lubani Al Saleh Teebi syndrome
— Lubinsky syndrome
— Lucey Driscoll syndrome
— Lucky Gelehrter syndrome
— Lúes Congénita

- Luiphobia
- Lujan-Fryns syndrome
- Lumbar malsegmentation short stature
- Lundberg syndrome
- Lung agenesis heart defect thumb anomalies
- Lung cancer
- Lung herniation congenital defect of sternem
- Lung neoplasm
- Lupus anticoagulant, familial
- Lupus erythematosus
- Lurie Kletsky syndrome
- Luteinizing hormone releasing hormone, deficiency of with ataxia
- Lutz Richner Landolt syndrome
- Lutz-Lewandowsky epidermodysplasia verruciformis
- Lyell's syndrome
- Lygophobia
- Lyme disease
- Lymph node neoplasm
- Lymphadenopathy, angioimmunoblastic with dysproteinemia
- Lymphangiectasies lymphoedema type Hennekam type
- Lymphangiectasis
- Lymphangioleiomyomatosis
- Lymphangiomatosis, pulmonary
- Lymphangiomyomatosis
- Lymphatic filariasis
- Lymphatic neoplasm
- Lymphedema distichiasis
- Lymphedema hereditary type 1
- Lymphedema hereditary type 2
- Lymphedema ptosis
- Lymphedema, congenital
- Lymphedema
- Lymphedema-Distichiasis syndrome
- Lymphoblastic lymphoma
- Lymphocytes reduced or absent
- Lymphocytic colitis
- Lymphocytic infiltrate of Jessner
- Lymphocytic vasculitis
- Lymphoid hamartoma

— Lymphoma, AIDS-related
— Lymphoma, gastric non Hodgkins type
— Lymphoma, large-cell, immunoblastic
— Lymphoma, large-cell
— Lymphoma, small cleaved-cell, diffuse
— Lymphoma, small cleaved-cell, follicular
— Lymphoma
— Lymphomatoid granulomatosis
— Lymphomatoid papulosis (LyP)
— Lymphomatous thyroiditis
— Lymphosarcoma
— Lynch Lee Murday syndrome
— Lynch-Bushby syndrome
— Lyngstadaas syndrome
— LyP (lymphomatoid papulosis)
— Lysine alpha-ketoglutarate reductase deficiency
— Lysinuric protein intolerance
— Lysosomal alpha-D-mannosidase deficiency
— Lysosomal beta-mannosidase deficiency
— Lysosomal disorders
— Lysosomal glycogen storage disease with normal acid maltase activity

M

— Mac Ardle disease
— Mac Dermot Patton Williams syndrome
— Mac Dermot Winter syndrome
— Macias Flores Garcia Cruz Rivera syndrome
— Mackay Shek Carr syndrome
— Macleod Fraser syndrome
— Macrocephaly cutis marmorata telangiectatica
— Macrocephaly dominant type
— Macrocephaly mental retardation facial dysmorphism
— Macrocephaly mesodermal hamartoma spectrum
— Macrocephaly mesomelic arms talipes
— Macrocephaly pigmentation large hands feet
— Macrocephaly short stature paraplegia
— Macrodactyly of the foot
— Macrodactyly of the hand
— Macroepiphyseal dysplasia Mcalister Coe type

- — Macroglobulinemia
- — Macroglossia dominant
- — Macroglossia exomphalos gigantism
- — Macrogyria pseudobulbar palsy
- — Macrophagic myofasciitis
- — Macrosomia developmental delay dysmorphism
- — Macrosomia microphthalmia cleft palate
- — Macrothrombocytopenia progressive deafness
- — Macrothrombocytopenia with leukocyte inclusions
- — Macular corneal dystrophy
- — Macular degeneration juvenile
- — Macular degeneration, age-related
- — Macular degeneration, polymorphic
- — Macular degeneration
- — Macular dystrophy, vitelliform
- — Macules hereditary congenital hypopigmented and hyperpigmented
- — Mad cow disease
- — Madelung's disease
- — Madokoro Ohdo Sonoda syndrome
- — Maffucci syndrome
- — Mageirocophobia
- — Maghazaji syndrome
- — Magnesium defect in renal tubular transport of
- — Magnesium wasting renal
- — Mal de debarquement
- — Malakoplakia
- — Malaria
- — Male pseudohermaphroditism due to 17-beta-hydroxysteroid dehydrogenase deficiency
- — Male pseudohermaphroditism due to 5-alpha-reductase 2 deficiency
- — Male pseudohermaphroditism due to defective LH molecule
- — Malformations in neuronal migration
- — Malignant astrocytoma
- — Malignant fibrous histiocytoma
- — Malignant germ cell tumor
- — Malignant hyperthermia arthrogryposis torticollis
- — Malignant hyperthermia
- — Malignant mesenchymal tumor

— Malignant mixed Mullerian tumor
— Malignant paroxysmal ventricular tachycardia
— Mallory-Weiss syndrome
— Malonic aciduria
— Malonyl-CoA decarboxylase deficiency
— Malouf syndrome
— Malpuech facial clefting syndrome
— Mandibuloacral dysplasia
— Mandibulofacial dysostosis deafness postaxial polydactly
— Manic Depression, Bipolar
— Manic-depressive psychosis, genetic types
— Mannosidosis
— Manouvrier syndrome
— Mansonelliasis
— Mantle cell lymphoma
— Marashi Gorlin syndrome
— Marburg fever
— Marchiafava Bignami disease
— Marchiafava-Micheli disease
— Marcus Gunn phenomenon
— Marden Walker like syndrome
— Marden-Walker syndrome
— Marek disease
— Marfan Syndrome type II
— Marfan Syndrome type III
— Marfan Syndrome type IV
— Marfan Syndrome type V
— Marfan syndrome
— Marfan-like syndrome, Boileau type
— Marfan-Like syndrome
— Marfanoid craniosynostosis syndrome
— Marfanoid hypermobility
— Marfanoid mental retardation syndrome autosomal
— Marginal glioneuronal heterotopia
— Marie type ataxia
— Marie Unna congenital hypotrichosis
— Marinesco Sjogren like syndrome
— Marinesco-Sjogren syndrome
— Marion Mayers syndrome
— Markel Vikkula Mulliken syndrome

— Marles Greenberg Persaud syndrome
— Maroteaux Cohen Solal Bonaventure syndrome
— Maroteaux Fonfria syndrome
— Maroteaux Le Merrer Bensahel syndrome
— Maroteaux Stanescu Cousin syndrome
— Maroteaux Verloes Stanescu syndrome
— Maroteaux-Lamy syndrome
— Marphanoid syndrome type De Silva
— Marsden Nyhan Sakati syndrome
— Marsden syndrome
— Marshall syndrome
— Marshall-Smith syndrome
— Martinez Monasterio Pinheiro syndrome
— Martsolf Reed Hunter syndrome
— Martsolf syndrome
— MASA syndrome
— Mass syndrome
— Massa Casaer Ceulemans syndrome
— Mast cell disease
— Mastigophobia
— Mastocytosis, short stature, hearing loss
— Mastocytosis
— Mastoiditis
— Mastroiacovo De Rosa Satta syndrome
— Mastroiacovo Gambi Segni syndrome
— MAT deficiency
— Maternal hyperphenylalaninemia
— Maternally inherited diabetes and deafness
— Mathieu De Broca Bony syndrome
— Matsoukas Liarikos Giannika syndrome
— Matthew-Wood syndrome
— Maturity onset diabetes of the young
— Maumenee syndrome
— Maxillary double lip
— Maxillofacial dysostosis
— Maxillonasal dysplasia, Binder type
— Mayer Rokitanski Kuster syndrome
— May-Hegglin Anomaly
— McAlister Crane syndrome
— McArdle disease

— McCallum Macadam Johnston syndrome
— McCune-Albright syndrome
— McDonough syndrome
— McDowall syndrome
— McGillivray syndrome
— McKusick Kaufman syndrome
— McKusick type metaphyseal chondrodysplasia
— McLain Debakian syndrome
— McPherson Clemens syndrome
— McPherson Robertson Cammarano syndrome
— Meacham Winn Culler syndrome
— Meadows syndrome
— Measles
— Meckel like syndrome
— Meckel syndrome
— Medeira Dennis Donnai syndrome
— Median cleft lip corpus callosum lipoma skin polyps
— Median nodule of the upper lip
— Mediastinal endodermal sinus tumors
— Mediterranean fever
— Medium-chain Acyl-CoA dehydrogenase deficiency
— Medrano Roldan syndrome
— Medullary cystic disease
— Medullary thyroid carcinoma
— Medulloblastoma
— Megacystis microcolon intestinal hypoperistalsis syndrome
— Megaduodenum
— Megaepiphyseal dwarfism
— Megalencephalic leukodystrophy
— Megalencephaly-cystic leukodystrophy
— Megaloblastic anemia
— Megalocornea mental retardation syndrome
— Megalocytic Interstitial Nephritis
— Mehes syndrome
— Mehta Lewis Patton syndrome
— Meier Blumberg Imahorn syndrome
— Meier Rotschild syndrome
— Meige syndrome
— Meigel disease
— Meinecke Pepper syndrome

— Meinecke syndrome
— Melanoma type 1
— Melanoma type 2
— Melanoma, familial
— Melanoma, Malignant
— Melanoma-astrocytoma syndrome
— Melanosis neurocutaneous
— MELAS
— Meleda Disease
— Melhem Fahl syndrome
— Melioidosis
— Melkersson-Rosenthal syndrome
— Melnick-Needles osteodysplasty
— Melnick-Needles syndrome
— Melophobia
— Membranoproliferative glomerulonephritis (type II)
— Mendelian susceptibility to atypical mycobacteria
— Menetrier's disease
— Mengel Konigsmark syndrome
— Ménière's disease
— Meningeal angiomatosis cleft hypoplastic left heart
— Meningioma 1
— Meningioma
— Meningitis, meningococcal
— Meningitis
— Meningocele
— Meningococcemia
— Meningoencephalocele
— Mental retardation athetosis microphthalmia
— Mental retardation blepharophimosis obesity web neck
— Mental retardation Buenos Aires type
— Mental retardation cataracts calcified pinnae myopathy
— Mental retardation coloboma slimness
— Mental retardation contractural arachnodactyly
— Mental retardation dysmorphism hypogonadism diabetes
— Mental retardation epilepsy bulbous nose
— Mental retardation epilepsy
— Mental retardation gynecomastia obesity X linked
— Mental retardation hip luxation G6PD variant
— Mental retardation hypocupremia hypobetalipoproteinemia

— Mental retardation hypotonia skin hyperpigmentation
— Mental retardation macrocephaly coarse facies hypotonia
— Mental retardation microcephaly phalangeal facial
— Mental retardation microcephaly unusual facies
— Mental retardation Mietens Weber type
— Mental retardation multiple nevi
— Mental retardation myopathy short stature endocrine defect
— Mental retardation nasal hypoplasia obesity genital hypoplasia
— Mental retardation nasal papillomata
— Mental retardation osteosclerosis
— Mental retardation progressive spasticity
— Mental retardation psychosis macroorchidism
— Mental retardation short broad thumbs
— Mental retardation short stature absent phalanges
— Mental retardation short stature Bombay phenotype
— Mental retardation short stature cleft palate unusual facies
— Mental retardation short stature deafness genital
— Mental retardation short stature hand contractures genital anomalies
— Mental retardation short stature heart and skeletal anomalies
— Mental retardation short stature hypertelorism
— Mental retardation short stature microcephaly eye
— Mental retardation short stature ocular and articular anomalies
— Mental retardation short stature scoliosis
— Mental retardation short stature unusual facies
— Mental retardation short stature wedge shaped epiphyses
— Mental retardation unusual facies Davis Lafer type
— Mental retardation unusual facies talipes hand anomalies
— Mental retardation unusual facies
— Mental retardation Wolff type
— Mental retardation X linked Atkin type
— Mental retardation
— Mental retardation-polydactyly-uncombable hair
— Mercury poisoning
— Meretoja syndrome
— Merkle tumors
— Merlob Grunebaum Reisner syndrome
— Merlob syndrome
— Mesangial sclerosis, diffuse

- Mesenteric ischemia
- Mesenteric panniculitis
- Mesodermal defects lower type
- Mesomelia synostoses
- Mesomelia
- Mesomelic dwarfism cleft palate camptodactyly
- Mesomelic dwarfism Langer type
- Mesomelic dwarfism Nievergelt type
- Mesomelic dwarfism Reinhardt Pfeiffer type
- Mesomelic dysplasia skin dimples
- Mesomelic dysplasia Thai type
- Mesomelic syndrome Pfeiffer type
- Mesothelioma
- Metabolic acidosis
- Metabolic disorder
- Metabolic Syndrome X
- Metacarpals 4 and 5 fusion
- Metachondromatosis
- Metageria
- Metaphyseal anadysplasia
- Metaphyseal chondrodysplasia Schmid type
- Metaphyseal chondrodysplasia Spahr type
- Metaphyseal chondrodysplasia, others
- Metaphyseal dysostosis mental retardation conductive deafness
- Metaphyseal dysplasia maxillary hypoplasia brachydactyly
- Metaphyseal dysplasia Pyle type
- Metastatic insulinoma
- Metatarsus adductus
- Metathesiophobia
- Metatrophic dysplasia
- Metatropic dwarfism
- Methimazole antenatal infection
- Methionine adenosyl transferase deficiency
- Methyl mercury antenatal infection
- Methylcobalamin deficiency cbl G type
- Methylcobalamin deficiency, cbl E complementation type
- Methylenetetrahydrofolate reductase deficiency
- Methylmalonic acidemia with homocystinuria
- Methylmalonic acidemia
- Methylmalonic aciduria microcephaly cataract

— Methylmalonicacidemia with homocystinuria, cbl D
— Methylmalonicaciduria with homocystinuria, cbl F
— Methylmalonicaciduria, vitamin B12 unresponsive, mut-0
— Methylmalonyl-Coenzyme A mutase deficiency
— Mevalonate kinase deficiency
— Mevalonicaciduria
— Meyenburg-Altherr-Uehlinger syndrome
— Michelin tire baby syndrome
— Michels Caskey syndrome
— Michels syndrome
— Mickleson syndrome
— Micrencephaly corpus callosum agenesis
— Micrencephaly olivopontocerebellar hypoplasia
— Micro syndrome
— Microcephaly autosomal dominant
— Microcephaly brachydactyly kyphoscoliosis
— Microcephaly brain defect spasticity hypernatremia
— Microcephaly cardiac defect lung malsegmentation
— Microcephaly cardiomyopathy
— Microcephaly cervical spine fusion anomalies
— Microcephaly chorioretinopathy recessive form
— Microcephaly cleft palate autosomal dominant
— Microcephaly deafness syndrome
— Microcephaly developmental delay pancytopenia
— Microcephaly facial clefting preaxial polydactyly
— Microcephaly glomerulonephritis Marfanoid habitus
— Microcephaly hiatus hernia nephrotic syndrome
— Microcephaly hypergonadotropic hypogonadism short stature
— Microcephaly immunodeficiency lymphoreticuloma
— Microcephaly intracranial calcification
— Microcephaly nonsyndromal
— Microcephaly pontocerebellar hypoplasia dyskinesia
— Microcephaly seizures mental retardation heart disorders
— Microcephaly sparse hair mental retardation seizures
— Microcephaly syndactyly brachymesophalangy
— Microcephaly with chorioretinopathy, autosomal dominant form
— Microcephaly with normal intelligence, immunodeficiency
— Microcephaly with spastic quadriplegia
— Microgastria short stature diabetes
— Microinfarct

— Micromelic dwarfism Fryns type
— Micromelic dysplasia dislocation of radius
— Microphobia
— Microphtalmos bilateral colobomatous orbital cyst
— Microphthalmia camptodactyly mental retardation
— Microphthalmia cataract
— Microphthalmia diaphragmatic hernia Fallot
— Microphthalmia mental deficiency
— Microphthalmia microtia fetal akinesia
— Microphthalmia, Lentz type
— Microphthalmia
— Microphthalmos, microcornea, and sclerocornea
— Microscopic polyangiitis
— Microsomia hemifacial radial defects
— Microspherophakia metaphyseal dysplasia
— Microsporidiosis
— Microtia, meatal atresia and conductive deafness
— Microvillus inclusion disease
— Miculicz syndrome
— MIDAS syndrome
— Midline cleft of lower lip
— Midline defects autosomal type
— Midline defects recessive type
— Midline developmental field defects
— Midline field defects
— Midline lethal granuloma
— Mietens syndrome
— Mievis Verellen Dumoulin syndrome
— Migraine
— Mikulicz' Disease
— Mikulicz syndrome
— Miller Fisher syndrome
— Miller-Dieker syndrome
— Milner Khallouf Gibson syndrome
— MILS syndrome
— Minkowski-Chauffard disease
— Minoxidil antenatal infection
— Miosis, congenital
— Mirror hands feet nasal defects
— Mirror polydactyly segmentation and limbs defects

— Misophobia
— Mitochondrial cytopathy (generic term)
— Mitochondrial diseases of nuclear origin
— Mitochondrial diseases, clinically undefinite
— Mitochondrial Diseases
— Mitochondrial encephalomyopathy aminoacidopathy
— Mitochondrial genetic disorders
— Mitochondrial myopathy lactic acidosis
— Mitochondrial myopathy-encephalopathy-lactic acidosis
— Mitochondrial PEPCK deficiency
— Mitochondrial trifunctional protein deficiency
— Mitral atresia
— Mitral regurgitation deafness skeletal anomalies
— Mitral valve prolapse, familial, autosomal dominant
— Mitral valve prolapse, familial, X linked
— Mitral valve prolapse
— Miura syndrome
— Mixed connective tissue disease
— Mixed Mullerian tumor
— Mixed sclerosing bone dystrophy
— MLS syndrome
— MMEP syndrome
— MMT syndrome
— MN1
— MNGIE syndrome
— Mobius syndrome
— MODY syndrome
— Moebius axonal neuropathy hypogonadism
— Moebius syndrome
— Moerman Van den berghe Fryns syndrome
— Moeschler Clarren syndrome
— Mohr syndrome
— Mohr-Tranebjaerg syndrome
— Mollica Pavone Antener syndrome
— Molluscum contagiosum
— Moloney syndrome
— Molybdenum cofactor deficiency
— MOMO syndrome
— Mondini Dysplasia
— Mondor's disease

— Monge's disease
— Monilethrix
— Monoamine oxidase A deficiency
— Monoclonal gammopathy of undetermined significance
— Monodactyly tetramelic
— Mononen Karnes Senac syndrome
— Mononeuritis multiplex
— Monosomy 8q12 21
— Monosomy 8q21 q22
— Monosomy X
— Montefiore syndrome
— Moore Federman syndrome
— Moore Smith Weaver syndrome
— Morel's ear
— Moreno Zachai Kaufman syndrome
— Morgani Turner Albright syndrome
— Morhosseini Holmes Walton syndrome
— Morillo Cucci Passarge syndrome
— Morphea Scleroderma
— Morphea, generalized
— Morquio disease, type A
— Morquio disease, type B
— Morquio syndrome
— Morrison Young syndrome
— Morse Rawnsley Sargent syndrome
— Motor neuron disease
— Motor neuro-ophthalmic disorders
— Motor neuropathy peripheral dysautonomia
— Motor neuropathy
— Motor sensory neuropathy type 1 aplasia cutis congenita
— Mounier-Kuhn syndrome
— Mount Reback syndrome
— Mousa Al din Al Nassar syndrome
— Moyamoya disease
— MPO deficiency
— MPS III-A
— MPS III-B
— MPS III-C
— MPS III-D
— MPS VI

— MRKH Syndrome (Mullerian Agenesis)
— MSBD syndrome
— MTHFR deficiency
— Mucha-Habermann disease
— Muckle-Wells syndrome
— Mucoepithelial dysplasia
— Mucolipidosis type 1
— Mucolipidosis type 3
— Mucolipidosis type 4
— Mucopolysaccharidosis type 3
— Mucopolysaccharidosis type 4
— Mucopolysaccharidosis
— Mucosulfatidosis
— Muenke Syndrome
— Mulibrey Nanism syndrome
— Muller Barth Menger syndrome
— Mullerian agenesis
— Mullerian aplasia
— Mullerian derivatives lymphangiectasia polydactyly
— Mullerian derivatives, persistent
— Mullerian duct abnormalities galactosemia
— Mulliez Roux Loterman syndrome
— Multicentric osteolysis nephropathy
— Multicentric reticulohistiocytosis
— Multiple carboxylase deficiency, late onset
— Multiple carboxylase deficiency, propionic acidemia
— Multiple chemical sensitivity
— Multiple congenital anomalies mental retardation, growth failure and cleft lip palate
— Multiple congenital contractures
— Multiple contracture syndrome Finnish type
— Multiple endocrine neoplasia type
— Multiple fibrofolliculoma familial
— Multiple hereditary exostoses
— Multiple joint dislocations metaphyseal dysplasia
— Multiple myeloma
— Multiple organ failure
— Multiple pterygium syndrome lethal type
— Multiple sclerosis
— Multiple subcutaneous angiolipomas

— Multiple sulfatase deficiency
— Multiple synostoses syndrome 1
— Multiple system atrophy
— Multiple vertebral anomalies unusual facies
— Mumps
— Munchausen by proxy syndrome
— Muscle-eye-brain syndrome
— Muscular atrophy ataxia retinitis pigmentosa diabetes mellitus
— Muscular dystrophy congenital infantile cataract hypogonadism
— Muscular dystrophy congenital, merosin negative
— Muscular dystrophy facioscapulohumeral
— Muscular dystrophy Hutterite type
— Muscular dystrophy limb girdle type 2A, Erb type
— Muscular dystrophy limb-girdle autosomal dominant
— Muscular dystrophy limb-girdle type 2B, Myoshi type
— Muscular dystrophy limb-girdle with beta-sarcoglycan deficiency
— Muscular dystrophy limb-girdle with delta-sarcoglyan deficiency
— Muscular dystrophy white matter spongiosis
— Muscular dystrophy, congenital, merosin-positive
— Muscular dystrophy, Duchenne and Becker type
— Muscular dystrophy
— Muscular fibrosis multifocal obstructed vessels
— Muscular phosphorylase kinase deficiency
— Mutations in estradiol receptor
— Myalgia eosinophilia associated with tryptophan
— Myalgic encephalomyelitis
— Myasthenia gravis congenital
— Myasthenia gravis
— Myasthenia, familial
— Mycetoma
— Mycobacterium avium complex infection
— Mycophobia
— Mycoplasmal pneumonia
— Mycosis fungoides lymphoma
— Mycosis fungoides, familial
— Mycosis fungoides
— Mycositis fungoides
— Myelinopathies
— Myelitis
— Myelocerebellar disorder

— Myelodysplasia
— Myelodysplastic syndromes
— Myelofibrosis, idiopathic
— Myelofibrosis
— Myelofibrosis-osteosclerosis
— Myeloid splenomegaly
— Myeloperoxidase deficiency
— Myhre Ruvalcaba Graham syndrome
— Myhre Ruvalcaba Kelley syndrome
— Myhre School syndrome
— Myhre syndrome
— Myiasis
— Myoadenylate deaminase deficiency
— Myocarditis
— Myocardium disorder
— Myoclonic dystonia
— Myoclonic progressive familial epilepsy
— Myoclonus ataxia
— Myoclonus cerebellar ataxia deafness
— Myoclonus epilepsy partial seizure
— Myoclonus epilepsy
— Myoclonus hereditary progressive distal muscular atrophy
— Myoclonus progressive epilepsy of Unverricht and Lundborg
— Myoclonus with epilepsy with ragged red fibers (mitochondria)
— Myoclonus
— Myofibrillar lysis
— Myofibroblastic tumors
— Myoglobinuria dominant form
— Myoglobinuria recurrent
— Myoglobinuria
— Myoneurogastrointestinal encephalopathy syndrome
— Myopathy and diabetes mellitus
— Myopathy cataract hypogonadism
— Myopathy congenital multicore with external ophthalmoplegia
— Myopathy growth and mental retardation hypospadias
— Myopathy Hutterite type
— Myopathy mitochondrial cataract
— Myopathy Moebius Robin syndrome
— Myopathy ophthalmoplegia hypoacousia areflexia
— Myopathy tubular aggregates

— Myopathy with lactic acidosis and sideroblastic anemia
— Myopathy with lysis of myofibrils
— Myopathy, centronuclear
— Myopathy, desmin storage
— Myopathy, McArdle type
— Myopathy, myotubular
— Myopathy, X-linked, with excessive autophagy
— Myopathy
— Myophosphorylase deficiency
— Myopia
— Myopia, infantile severe
— Myopia, severe
— Myotubular myopathy
— Myositis ossificans post-traumatic
— Myositis ossificans progressiva
— Myositis ossificans
— Myositis, inclusion body
— Myositis
— Myotonia atrophica
— Myotonia mental retardation skeletal anomalies
— Myxedema
— Myxoma-spotty pigmentation-endocrine overactivity
— Myxomatous peritonitis
— N syndrome
— N-acetyl glutamate synthetase deficiency
— N-acetyl-alpha-D-galactosaminidase
— N-acetyl-glucosamine-6-sulfate sulfatase deficiency
— NADH CoQ reductase, deficiency of
— NADH cytochrome B5 reductase deficiency
— Naegeli syndrome
— Naguib syndrome
— Nail-patella syndrome
— Nakajo Nishimura syndrome
— Nakajo syndrome
— Nakamura Osame syndrome
— NAME syndrome
— Nance-Horan syndrome
— Nanism due to growth hormone combined deficiency
— Nanism due to growth hormone isolated deficiency with X linked hypogammaglobulinemia

— Nanism due to growth hormone resistance
— Narcolepsy
— Narcolepsy-Cataplexy
— Narrow oral fissure short stature cone shaped epiphyses
— Nasodigitoacoustic syndrome
— Nasopalpebral lipoma coloboma syndrome
— Nasopharyngeal carcinoma
— Nasopharyngeal teratoma Dandy Walker diaphragmatic hernia
— Natal teeth intestinal pseudoobstruction patent ductus
— Nathalie syndrome
— Native American myopathy
— Navajo poikiloderma
— Naxos disease
— Necrotizing encephalopathy, infantile subacute
— Necrotizing fasciitis
— Negative rheumatoid factor polyarthritis
— Neisseria meningitidis
— Nelson syndrome
— Nemaline myopathy
— Nemaline Myopathy, Amish Type
— Neonatal hemochromatosis
— Neonatal hepatitis
— Neonatal herpes
— Neonatal ovarian cyst
— Neonatal transient jaundice
— Neopharmaphobia
— Nephroblastomatosis,fetal ascites,macrosomia and Wilm's tumor
— Nephrocalcinosis
— Nephrogenic diabetes insipidus
— Nephrolithiasis type 2
— Nephronophthisis familial adult spastic quadriparesis
— Nephropathy deafness hyperparathyroidism
— Nephropathy familial with hyperuricemia
— Nephropathy, familial with gout
— Nephrosclerosis
— Nephrosis deafness urinary tract digital malformation
— Nephrosis neuronal dysmigration syndrome
— Nephrotic syndrome
— Nephrotic syndrome ocular anomalies
— Nephrotic syndrome, idiopathic, steroid-resistant

— Nerve sheath neoplasm
— Nesidioblastosis of pancreas
— Netherton syndrome ichthyosis
— Neu Laxova syndrome
— Neuhauser Daly Magnelli syndrome
— Neuhauser Eichner Opitz syndrome
— Neural crest tumor
— Neural tube defect, folate-sensitive
— Neural tube defects X linked
— Neuraminidase beta-galactosidase deficiency
— Neuraminidase deficiency
— Neurasthenia
— Neurilemmomatosis
— Neuritis with brachial predilection
— Neuroacanthocytosis
— Neuroaxonal dystrophy renal tubular acidosis
— Neuroaxonal dystrophy, late infantile
— Neuroblastoma
— Neurocutaneous melanosis
— Neuroectodermal endocrine syndrome
— Neuroectodermal tumors primitive
— Neuroendocrine cancer
— Neuroendocrine carcinoma of the cervix
— Neuroendocrine tumor
— Neuroepithelioma
— Neurofaciodigitorenal syndrome
— Neurofibrillary tangles
— Neurofibroma
— Neurofibromatosis
— Neurofibromatosis type 2
— Neurofibromatosis type 3
— Neurofibromatosis type 6
— Neurofibromatosis, familial intestinal
— Neurofibromatosis, Type IV, of Riccardi
— Neurofibromatosis-Noonan syndrome
— Neurofibrosarcoma
— Neurogenic hypertension
— Neuroleptic malignant syndrome
— Neuroma biliary tract
— Neuronal heterotopia

— Neuronal interstitial dysplasia
— Neuronal intestinal pseudoobstruction
— Neuronal intranuclear hyaline inclusion disease
— Neuronal intranuclear inclusion disease
— Neuropathy ataxia and retinis pigmentosa
— Neuropathy congenital sensory neurotrophic keratitis
— Neuropathy hereditary with liability to pressure palsies
— Neuropathy motor sensory type 2 deafness mental retardation
— Neuropathy sensory spastic paraplegia
— Neuropathy, hereditary motor and sensory, LOM type
— Neuropathy, hereditary sensory, type I
— Neuropathy, hereditary sensory, type II
— Neurotoxicity syndromes
— Neutral lipid storage myopathy
— Neutropenia intermittent
— Neutropenia monocytopenia deafness
— Neutropenia, severe chronic
— Nevi flammei, familial multiple
— Nevo syndrome
— Nevoid basal cell carcinoma syndrome
— Nevus of ota retinitis pigmentosa
— Nevus sebaceus of Jadassohn
— Nezelof's syndrome
— Nicolaides Baraitser syndrome
— Niemann-Pick C1 disease
— Niemann-Pick C2 disease
— Niemann-Pick disease type C
— Niemann-Pick disease type D
— Niemann-Pick Disease
— Night blindness skeletal anomalies unusual facies
— Night blindness, congenital stationary
— Nijmegen Breakage Syndrome
— Nivelon Nivelon Mabille syndrome
— Noble Bass Sherman syndrome
— Nocardiosis
— Noise induced deafness
— Nomá
— Non functioning pancreatic endocrine tumor
— Nonallergic atopic dermatitis
— Non-Hodgkin lymphoma

— Noninsulin-dependent diabetes mellitus with deafness
— Nonketotic hyperglycinemia
— Non-lissencephalic cortical dysplasia
— Nonmedullary thyroid carcinoma, with cell oxyphilia
— Nonne-Milroy disease
— Non-small cell lung cancer
— Nonsyndromic hereditary hearing impairment
— Noonan like syndrome
— Noonan syndrome
— Norman Roberts lissencephaly syndrome
— Normokalemic periodic paralysis
— Norrie disease
— Northern epilepsy
— Norum disease
— Nose polyposis, familial
— Nosocomephobia
— Notalgia paresthetica

O

— O Doherty syndrome
— O Donnell Pappas syndrome
— Obesity
— Obesophobia
— Obsessive-compulsive disorder
— Obstructive asymmetric septal hypertrophy
— Occipital horn syndrome
— Occlusive Infantile ateriopathy
— Occult spinal dysraphism
— Occupational Asthma - Chemicals
— Occupational Asthma - Metals
— Occupational Asthma - Plants
— Occupational Asthma - Wood dust
— Occupational Asthma-Drugs
— OCD
— Ochoa syndrome
— Ochronosis, hereditary
— Ochronosis
— Ockelbo disease
— Ocular Albinism
— Ocular coloboma-imperforate anus

— Ocular convergence spasm
— Ocular Histoplasmosis
— Ocular melanoma
— Ocular motility disorders
— Ocular toxoplasmosis
— Oculo cerebral dysplasia
— Oculo cerebro acral syndrome
— Oculo cerebro osseous syndrome
— Oculo dento digital dysplasia
— Oculo digital syndrome
— Oculo facio cardio dental syndrome
— Oculo skeletal renal syndrome
— Oculo tricho anal syndrome
— Oculo tricho dysplasia
— Oculoauriculofrontonasal syndrome
— Oculoauriculovertebral dysplasia
— Oculocerebral hypopigmentation syndrome Cross type
— Oculocerebral hypopigmentation syndrome type Preus
— Oculocerebral syndrome with hypopigmentation
— Oculocerebrocutaneous syndrome
— Oculocerebrorenal syndrome
— Oculocutaneous albinism immunodeficiency
— Oculocutaneous albinism type 1
— Oculocutaneous albinism type 2
— Oculocutaneous albinism type 3
— Oculocutaneous albinism, tyrosinase negative
— Oculocutaneous albinism, tyrosinase positive
— Oculocutaneous tyrosinemia
— Oculodental syndrome Rutherfurd syndrome
— Oculodentodigital dysplasia dominant
— Oculodentodigital syndrome
— Oculo-dento-digital syndrome
— Oculodentoosseous dysplasia dominant
— Oculodentoosseous dysplasia recessive
— Oculodigitoesophagoduodenal syndrome
— Oculo-gastrointestinal muscular dystrophy
— Oculomaxillofacial dysostosis
— Oculomaxillofacial dysplasia with oblique facial clefts
— Oculomelic amyoplasia
— Oculopalatoskeletal syndrome

— Oculopharyngeal muscular dystrophy
— Oculorenocerebellar syndrome
— Odonto onycho dysplasia with alopecia
— Odontoma
— Odontomicronychial dysplasia
— Odontoonychodermal dysplasia
— Odontophobia
— Odontotrichomelic hypohidrotic dysplasia
— Odynophobia
— OFD syndrome type 8
— OFD syndrome type Figuera
— Ogilvie's syndrome
— Ohaha syndrome
— Ohdo Madokoro Sonoda syndrome
— Oikophobia
— Okamuto Satomura syndrome
— Olfactophobia
— Oligodactyly
— Oligodactyly tetramelia postaxial
— Oligomeganephronic renal hypoplasia
— Oligomeganephrony
— Oligophernia
— Oliver McFarlane syndrome
— Oliver syndrome
— Olivopontocerebellar atrophy deafness
— Olivopontocerebellar atrophy type 1
— Olivopontocerebellar atrophy type 2
— Olivopontocerebellar atrophy type 3
— Olivopontocerebellar atrophy
— Ollier disease
— Olmsted syndrome
— Ombrophobia
— Omenn syndrome
— Omodysplasia type 1
— Omphalocele cleft palate syndrome lethal
— Omphalocele exstrophy imperforate anus
— Omphalomesenteric cyst
— Omsk hemorrhagic fever
— Onat syndrome
— Onchocerciasis

— Oncocytoma
— Ondine's curse
— Oneirophobia
— Onychonychia hypoplastic distal phalanges
— Onychotrichodysplasia and neutropenia
— Ophthalmic icthyosis
— Ophthalmo acromelic syndrome
— Ophthalmomandibulomelic dysplasia
— Ophthalmophobia
— Ophthalmoplegia ataxia hypoacusis
— Ophthalmoplegia mental retardation lingua scrotalis
— Ophthalmoplegia myalgia tubular aggregates
— Opitz Mollica Sorge syndrome
— Opitz Reynolds Fitzgerald syndrome
— Opitz syndrome
— Opportunistic infections
— Oppositional defiant disorder
— Opsismodysplasia
— Opthalmoplegia progressive external scoliosis
— Optic atrophy opthalmoplegia ptosis deafness myopia
— Optic atrophy polyneuropathy deafness
— Optic atrophy, autosomal dominant
— Optic atrophy, idiopathic, autosomal recessive
— Optic atrophy
— Optic nerve coloboma with renal disease
— Optic nerve disorder
— Optic nerve hypoplasia, familial bilateral
— Optic neuritis
— Optic pathway glioma
— Opticoacoustic nerve atrophy dementia
— Oral facial digital syndrome type 3
— Oral facial digital syndrome type 4
— Oral facial digital syndrome
— Oral facial dyskinesia
— Oral leukoplakia
— Oral lichen planus
— Oral lichenoid lesions
— Oral squamous cell carcinoma
— Oral submucous fibrosis
— Oral-facial cleft

— Oral-facial-digital syndrome, type IV
— Oral-facial-digital syndrome
— Oral-pharyngeal disorders
— Organic brain syndrome
— Organic mood syndrome
— Organic personality syndrome
— Ornithine aminotransferase deficiency
— Ornithine carbamoyl phosphate deficiency
— Ornithine transcarbamylase deficiency, hyperammonemia due to
— Ornithinemia
— Ornithosis
— Oro acral syndrome
— Orofaciodigital syndrome Gabrielli type
— Orofaciodigital syndrome Shashi type
— Orofaciodigital syndrome Thurston type
— Orofaciodigital syndrome type 2
— Orofaciodigital syndrome type1
— Orotic aciduria hereditary
— Orotic aciduria purines-pyrimidines
— Orotidylic decarboxylase deficiency
— Orstavik Lindemann Solberg syndrome
— Orthostatic intolerance
— Osebold Remondini syndrome
— Osgood-Schlatter disease
— Oslam syndrome
— Osmed Syndrome
— Ossicular Malformations, familial
— Osteitis deformans
— osteo: bone
— Osteoarthritis
— Osteoarthropathy of fingers familial
— Osteochondritis deformans juvenile
— Osteochondritis dissecans
— Osteochondritis
— Osteochondrodysplasia thrombocytopenia hydroce-phalus
— Osteochondroma
— Osteocraniostenosis
— Osteodysplasia familial Anderson type
— Osteodysplastic dwarfism Corsello type

— Osteoectasia familial
— Osteogenesis Imperfecta
— Osteogenesis imperfecta congenita microcephaly and cataracts
— Osteogenesis imperfecta congenital joint contractures
— Osteogenesis imperfecta retinopathy
— Osteogenic sarcoma
— Osteoglophonic dwarfism
— Osteolysis hereditary multicentric
— Osteolysis syndrome recessive
— Osteomalacia
— osteomyelitis
— Osteonecrosis
— Osteopathia condensans disseminata with osteopoikilosis
— Osteopathia striata cranial sclerosis
— Osteopathia striata pigmentary dermopathy white forelock
— Osteopetrosis autosomal dominant type 1
— Osteopetrosis lethal
— Osteopetrosis renal tubular acidosis
— Osteopetrosis, (generic term)
— Osteopetrosis, malignant
— Osteopetrosis, mild autosomal recessive form
— Osteopoikilosis
— Osteoporosis macrocephaly mental retardation blindness
— Osteoporosis oculocutaneous hypopigmentation syndrome
— Osteoporosis pseudoglioma syndrome
— osteoporosis
— Osteosarcoma limb anomalies erythroid macrocytosis
— Osteosclerose type Stanescu
— Osteosclerosis abnormalities of nervous system and meninges
— Osteosclerosis autosomal dominant Worth type
— Osteosclerosis
— Ostertag type amyloidosis
— Ota Kawamura Ito syndrome
— Oto palato digital syndrome type I and II
— Otodental dysplasia
— Otofaciocervical syndrome
— Otoonychoperoneal syndrome
— Oto-Palatal-digital syndrome
— Otopalatodigital syndrome type 2
— Otosclerosis, familial

— otosclerosis
— Otospondylomegaepiphyseal dysplasia
— Ouvrier Billson syndrome
— Ovarian cancer
— Ovarian carcinosarcoma
— Ovarian dwarfism as part of Turner Syndrome
— Ovarian dwarfism
— Ovarian insufficiency due to FSH resistance
— ovarian remnant syndrome
— Overfolded helix
— Overgrowth radial ray defect arthrogryposis
— Overgrowth syndrome type Fryer
— Overhydrated hereditary stomatocytosis
— Oxalosis

P

— Pachydermoperiostosis
— Pachygyria
— Pachyonychia congenita Jackson Lawler type
— Pacman syndrome
— Paes Whelan Modi syndrome
— Paget disease extramammary
— Paget disease juvenile type
— Paget's disease of bone
— Paget's disease of the breast
— Paget's disease, type 1
— Pagon Bird Detter syndrome
— Pagon Stephan syndrome
— Pai Levkoff syndrome
— Palant cleft palate syndrome
— Palindromic rheumatism
— Pallister-Hall syndrome
— Pallister-Killian syndrome
— Palmer Pagon syndrome
— Palmitoyl-protein thioesterase deficiency
— Palmoplantar Keratoderma
— Palmoplantar porokeratosis of Mantoux
— Palsy cerebral
— Pancreas agenesis
— Pancreas divisum

— Pancreatic adenoma
— Pancreatic beta cell agenesis with neonatal diabetes mellitus
— Pancreatic cancer
— Pancreatic carcinoma, familial
— Pancreatic diseases
— Pancreatic islet cell neoplasm
— Pancreatic islet cell tumors
— Pancreatic lipomatosis duodenal stenosis
— Pancreatitis, hereditary
— Pancreatoblastoma
— PANDAS
— Panhypopituitarism
— Panic disorder
— Panmyelophthisis aplastic anemia
— Panniculitis
— Panophobia
— Panostotic fibrous dysplasia
— Panthophobia
— Papilledema
— Papillion-Lefevre syndrome
— Papillitis
— Papilloma of choroid plexus
— Papular mucinosis
— Papular urticaria
— Paracoccidioidomycosis
— Paraganglioma
— Parainfluenza virus type 3 antenatal infection
— Paramyotonia congenita of Von Eulenburg
— Paramyotonia congenita
— Paraneoplastic cerebellar degeneration
— Paraomphalocele
— Paraparesis amyotrophy of hands and feet
— Paraphilia
— Paraplegia
— Paraplegia-brachydactyly-cone shaped epiphysis
— Paraplegia-mental retardation-hyperkeratosis
— Parapsoriasis
— Parasitophobia
— Parastremmatic dwarfism
— Parathyroid cancer

— Parathyroid neoplasm
— Paratyphoid fever
— PARC syndrome
— Parenchymatous cortical degeneration of cerebellum
— Paris-Trousseau thrombopenia
— Parkes-Weber syndrome
— Parkinson's disease
— Parkinson dementia Steele type
— Parkinsonism early onset mental retardation
— Parkinsonism
— Parkinson's disease
— Paroxysmal cold hemoglobinuria
— Paroxysmal dystonic choreoathetosis
— Paroxysmal nocturnal hemoglobinuria
— Paroxysmal ventricular fibrillation
— Parry-Romberg syndrome
— Pars planitis
— Parsonage Turner syndrome
— Partial agenesis of corpus callosum
— Partial atrioventricular canal
— Partial deletion of Y
— Partial gigantism in context of NF
— Partial lissencephaly
— Partington Anderson syndrome
— Partington Mulley syndrome
— Parturiphobia
— Parvovirus antenatal infection
— Pascuel Castroviejo syndrome
— Patau syndrome
— Patel Bixler syndrome
— Patella aplasia, coxa vara, tarsal synostosis
— Patella hypoplasia mental retardation
— Patent ductus arteriosus familial
— Patent ductus arteriosus
— Pathophobia
— Patterson Lowry syndrome
— Patterson pseudoleprechaunism syndrome
— Patterson Stevenson syndrome
— Pauciarticular chronic arthritis
— Pavone Fiumara Rizzo syndrome

— Peanut Hypersensitivity
— Pearson's marrow/pancreas syndrome
— Pediatric T-cell leukemia
— Pediculosis
— Peeling skin syndrome ichthyosis
— PEHO syndrome
— Pelizaeus-Merzbacher brain sclerosis
— Pelizaeus-Merzbacher disease, recessive, acute infantile
— Pelizaeus-Merzbacher disease
— Pelizaeus-Merzbacher leukodystrophy
— Pellagra like syndrome
— Pellagrophobia
— Pelvic dysplasia arthrogryposis of lower limbs
— Pelvic inflammatory disease
— Pelvic lipomatosis
— Pelvic shoulder dysplasia
— Pemphigus and fogo selvagem
— Pemphigus foliaceus
— Pemphigus vulgaris, familial
— Pemphigus vulgaris
— Pemphigus
— Pena Shokeir syndrome
— Pendred syndrome
— Penis agenesia
— Penoscrotal transposition
— Penta X syndrome
— Pentalogy of Cantrell
— Pentosuria
— Penttinen-Aula syndrome
— PEPCK 1 deficiency
— PEPCK 2 deficiency
— PEPCK deficiency, mitochondrial
— Peptidic growth factors deficiency
— Periarteritis nodosa
— Pericardial constriction growth failure
— Phenylketonuria
— Phenylketonuric embryopathy
— Pheochromocytoma as part of NF
— Pheochromocytoma
— Philadelphia-negative chronic myeloid leukemia

— Phocomelia contractures absent thumb
— Phocomelia ectrodactyly deafness sinus arrhythmia
— Phocomelia Schinzel type
— Phocomelia syndrome
— Phocomelia thrombocytopenia encephalocele
— Phosphate diabetes
— Phosphoenolpyruvate carboxykinase 1 deficiency
— Phosphoenolpyruvate carboxykinase 2 deficiency
— Phosphoenolpyruvate carboxykinase deficiency
— Phosphoglucomutase deficiency type 1
— Phosphoglucomutase deficiency type 2
— Phosphoglucomutase deficiency type 3
— Phosphoglucomutase deficiency type 4
— Phosphoglucomutase deficiency
— Phosphoglycerate kinase 1 deficiency
— Phosphoglycerate kinase deficiency
— Phosphomannoisomerase deficiency
— Phosphoribosylpyrophosphate synthetase deficiency
— Photoaugliaphobia
— Photosensitive epilepsy
— Phthiriophobia
— Physical urticaria
— Phytanic acid oxidase deficiency
— PIBIDS syndrome
— Pica
— Picardi-Lassueur-Little syndrome
— Pick disease of the brain
— Pickardt syndrome
— Pie Torcido
— Piebald trait neurologic defects
— Piebaldism
— Piepkorn Karp Hickoc syndrome
— Pierre Marie cerbellar ataxia
— Pierre Robin sequence congenital heart defect talipes
— Pierre Robin sequence faciodigital anomaly
— Pierre Robin syndrome fetal chondrodysplasia
— Pierre Robin syndrome hyperphalangy clinodactyly
— Pierre Robin syndrome skeletal dysplasia polydactyly
— Pierre Robin's sequence
— Pigmentary retinopathy

— Pigment-dispersion syndrome
— Pigmented villonodular synovitis
— Pignata guarino syndrome
— Pili canulati
— Pili multigemini
— Pili torti developmental delay neurological abnormalities
— Pili torti nerve deafness
— Pili torti onychodysplasia
— Pili torti
— Pillay syndrome
— Pilo dento ungular dysplasia microcephaly
— Pilonidal cyst
— Pilotto syndrome
— Pinealoma
— Pinheiro Freire Maia Miranda syndrome
— Pinsky Di George Harley syndrome
— Pinta
— Pipecolic acidemia
— PIRA
— Pitt Hopkins syndrome
— Pitt-Rogers-Danks syndrome
— Pituitary dwarfism 1
— Pityriasis lichenoides chronica
— Pityriasis lichenoides et varioliformis acuta
— Pityriasis rubra pilaris
— Piussan Lenaerts Mathieu syndrome
— Placenta disorder
— Placenta neoplasm
— Placental abruption
— Plagiocephaly X linked mental retardation
— Plague (bubonic, septicemic, pneumonic and pharyngeal)
— Plasmacytoma anaplastic
— Plasmalogenes synthesis deficiency isolated
— Plasminogen activitor inhibitor type 1 deficiency, congenital
— Plasminogen deficiency, congenital
— Platelet disorder
— Platyspondylic lethal chondrodysplasia
— Platyspondyly amelogenesis imperfecta
— Pleural effusion
— Pleuritis

— Pleuritis
— Plexosarcoma
— Plum syndrome
— Plummer-Vinson syndrome
— Pneumoconiosis
— Pneumocystis jiroveci pneumonia
— Pneumocystosis
— Pneumonia, eosinophilic
— Pneumothorax
— Podder-Tolmie syndrome
— POEMS syndrome
— Poedimus kyleopecia mental retardation
— Poikiloderma congenital with bullae Weary type
— Poikiloderma hereditary acrokeratotic Weary type
— Poikiloderma of Kindler
— Poikiloderma of Rothmund-Thomson
— Poikilodermatomyositis mental retardation
— Poikilodermia alopecia retrognathism cleft palate
— Pointer syndrome
— Poland syndrome
— Poliomyelitis (Polio)
— Poliosophobia
— Polyarteritis nodosa
— Polyarteritis
— Polyarthritis, systemic
— Polyarthritis
— Polychondritis
— Polycystic kidney disease, adult type
— Polycystic kidney disease, infantile type
— Polycystic kidney disease, infantile, type I
— Polycystic kidney disease, recessive type
— Polycystic kidney disease, type 1
— Polycystic kidney disease, type 2
— Polycystic kidney disease, type 3
— Polycystic kidney disease
— Polycystic ovarian disease, familial
— Polycystic ovarian syndrome
— Polycystic ovaries urethral sphincter dysfunction
— Polycythemia vera
— Polydactyly alopecia seborrheic dermatitis

— Polydactyly cleft lip palate psychomotor retardation
— Polydactyly myopia syndrome
— Polydactyly postaxial dental and vertebral
— Polydactyly postaxial with median cleft of upper lip
— Polydactyly postaxial
— Polydactyly preaxial type 1
— Polydactyly syndrome middle ray duplication
— Polydactyly visceral anomalies cleft lip palate
— Polydactyly
— Polyglucosan body disease, adult
— Polymicrogyria turricephaly hypogenitalism
— Polymorphic catecholergic ventricular tachycardia
— Polymorphic macular degeneration
— Polymorphous low-grade adenocarcinoma
— Polymyalgia rheumatica
— Polymyositis
— Polyneuritis
— Polyneuropathy hand defect
— Polyneuropathy mental retardation acromicria prema
— Polyomavirus Infections
— Polyostotic fibrous dysplasia
— Polyposis hamartomatous intestinal
— Polyposis skin pigmentation alopecia fingernail changes
— Polysyndactyly cardiac malformation
— Polysyndactyly microcephaly ptosis
— Polysyndactyly orofacial anomalies
— Polysyndactyly overgrowth syndrome
— Polysyndactyly trigonocephaly agenesis of corpus callosum
— Polysyndactyly type 4
— Polysyndactyly type Haas
— Pompe's disease
— Poncet-Spiegler's cylindroma
— Pontoneocerebellar Hypoplasia
— Popliteal pterygium syndrome lethal type
— Popliteal pterygium syndrome
— Porencephaly cerebellar hypoplasia malformations
— Porencephaly
— Porokeratosis of Mibelli
— Porokeratosis plantaris palmaris et disseminata
— Porokeratosis punctata palmaris et plantaris

— Porphyria
— Porphyria cutanea tarda, familial type
— Porphyria cutanea tarda, sporadic type
— Porphyria cutanea tarda
— Porphyria, acute intermittent
— Porphyria, Ala-D
— Porphyria, congenital erythropoietic
— Porphyria, hereditary coproporphyria
— Portal hypertension due to infrahepatic block
— Portal hypertension
— Portal thrombosis
— Portal vein thrombosis
— Portuguese type amyloidosis
— Positive rheumatoid factor polyarthritis
— Post Polio syndrome
— Post Traumatic Stress disorder (PTSD)
— Postaxial polydactyly mental retardation
— Posterior tibial tendon rupture
— Posterior urethral valves
— Posterior uveitis
— Posterior valve urethra
— Post-infectious myocarditis
— Post-traumatic epilepsy
— Postural hypotension
— Potassium aggravated myotonia
— Potassium deficiency (hypokalemia)
— Potter disease type 1
— Potter disease, type 3
— Potter sequence cleft cardiopathy
— Potter syndrome dominant type
— Powell Buist Stenzel syndrome
— Powell Chandra Saal syndrome
— Powell Venencie Gordon syndrome
— Poxviridae disease
— Prader-Willi syndrome
— Prata Liberal Goncalves syndrome
— Preaxial deficiency postaxial polydactyly hypospadia
— Preaxial polydactyly colobomata mental retardation
— Precocious epileptic encephalopathy
— Precocious myoclonic encephalopathy

— Precocious puberty, gonadotropin-dependent
— Precocious puberty, male limited
— Precocious puberty
— Preeclampsia
— Preeyasombat Viravithya syndrome
— Pregnancy toxemia /hypertension
— Prekallikrein deficiency, congenital
— Premature aging, Okamoto type
— Premature aging
— Premature atherosclerosis photomyoclonic epilepsy
— Premature menopause, familial
— Premature ovarian failure
— Premenstrual dysphoric disorder
— Prenatal infections
— Presbycusis
— Prieto Badia Mulas syndrome
— Prieur Griscelli syndrome
— Primary agammaglobulinemia
— Primary aldosteronism
— Primary alveolar hypoventilation
— Primary amenorrhea
— Primary biliary cirrhosis
— Primary ciliary dyskinesia, 2
— Primary ciliary dyskinesia
— Primary craniosynostosis
— Primary cutaneous amyloidosis
— Primary granulocytic sarcoma
— Primary hyperoxaluria
— Primary hyperparathyroidism
— Primary lateral sclerosis
— Primary malignant lymphoma
— Primary orthostatic tremor
— Primary progressive aphasia
— Primary pulmonary hypertension
— Primary sclerosing cholangitis
— Primary tubular proximal acidosis
— Primerose syndrome
— Primordial microcephalic dwarfism Crachami type
— Prinzmetal's variant angina
— Procarcinoma

— Proconvertin deficiency, congenital
— Proctitis
— Progeria short stature pigmented nevi
— Progeria variant syndrome Ruvalcaba type
— Progeria
— Progeroid syndrome De Barsy type
— Progeroid syndrome Petty type
— Progeroid syndrome, Penttinen type
— Prognathism dominant
— Progressive acromelanosis
— Progressive black carbon hyperpigmentation of infancy
— Progressive diaphyseal dysplasia
— Progressive external ophthalmoplegia
— Progressive hearing loss stapes fixation
— Progressive kinking of the hair, acquired
— Progressive multifocal leukoencephalopathy
— Progressive myositis ossificans
— Progressive osseous heteroplasia
— Progressive spinal muscular atrophy
— Progressive supranuclear palsy atypical
— Progressive supranuclear palsy
— Progressive systemic sclerosis
— Prolactinoma, familial
— Prolerating trichilemmal cyst
— Prolidase deficiency
— Prolymphocytic leukemia
— Properdin deficiency
— Prosencephaly cerebellar dysgenesis
— Prostaglandin antenatal infection
— Prostate cancer, familial
— Prostatic malacoplakia associated with prostatic abscess
— Prostatitis
— Protein C deficiency
— Protein-energy malnutrition
— Protein R deficiency
— Protein S acquired deficiency
— Protein S deficiency
— Proteus like syndrome mental retardation eye defect
— Proteus syndrome
— Prothrombin deficiency

— Protoporphyria, erythropoietic
— Protoporphyria
— Proud Levine Carpenter syndrome
— Proximal myotonic dystrophy
— Proximal myotonic myopathy
— Proximal spinal muscular atrophy
— Proximal tubulopathy diabetes mellitus cerebellar ataxia
— Pseudoachondroplastic dysplasia
— Pseudoadrenoleukodystrophy
— Pseudoaminopterin syndrome
— Pseudoarylsulfatase A deficiency
— Pseudocholinesterase deficiency
— Pseudo-Gaucher disease
— Pseudogout
— Pseudohermaphrodism anorectal anomalies
— Pseudohermaphroditism female skeletal anomalies
— Pseudohermaphroditism male with gynecomastia
— Pseudohermaphroditism mental retardation
— Pseudohermaphroditism
— Pseudohypoaldosteronism
— Pseudohypoaldosteronism
— Pseudohypoparathyroidism
— Pseudomarfanism
— Pseudopapilledema blepharophimosis hand anomalies
— Pseudo-Pelade of Brocq
— Pseudopolycythaemia
— Pseudoprogeria syndrome
— Pseudo-torch syndrome
— Pseudotumor cerebri
— Pseudo-Turner syndrome
— Pseudovaginal perineoscrotal hypospadias
— Pseudoxanthoma elasticum, dominant form
— Pseudoxanthoma elasticum, recessive form
— Pseudoxanthoma elasticum
— Pseudo-Zellweger syndrome
— Psittacosis
— Psoriasis
— Psoriatic arthritis
— Psoriatic rheumatism
— Psychogenic polydipsia

— Psychophysiologic Disorders
— Psychosis
— Pterigium Colli
— Pterygia mental retardation facial dysmorphism
— Pterygium colli mental retardation digital anomalies
— Pterygium of the conjunctiva
— Pterygium syndrome antecubital
— Pterygium syndrome multiple dominant type
— Pulmonary veins stenosis
— Pulmonary veno-occlusive disease
— Pulmonary venous return anomaly
— Pulmonaryatresia intact ventricular septum
— Pulmonic stenosis with Café au lait spot
— Punctate acrokeratoderma freckle like pigmentation
— Punctate inner choroidopathy
— Pupaphobia
— Pure red cell aplasia
— Puretic syndrome
— Purine nucleoside phosphorylase deficiency
— Purpura, Schoenlein-Henoch
— Purpura, thrombotic thrombocytopenic
— Purtilo syndrome
— Pyaemia
— Pycnodysostosis
— Pyknoachondrogenesis
— Pyle disease
— Pyelonephritis
— Pyoderma gangrenosum
— Pyomyositis
— Pyridoxine deficit
— Pyrimidinemia familial
— Pyrophobia
— Pyropoikilocytosis
— Pyrosis
— Pyruvate carboxylase deficiency
— Pyruvate decarboxylase deficiency
— Pyruvate dehydrogenase deficiency
— Pyruvate kinase deficiency, liver type
— Pyruvate kinase deficiency, muscle type
— Pyruvate kinase deficiency

Q

- Q fever
- Qazi Markouizos syndrome
- Quebec platelet disorder
- Quinquaud's decalvans folliculitis

R

- Rabies
- Rabson-Mendenhall syndrome
- Radial defect Robin sequence
- Radial hypoplasia, triphalangeal thumbs and hypospadias
- Radial ray agenesis
- Radial ray hypoplasia choanal atresia
- Radiation induced angiosarcoma of the breast
- Radiation induced meningioma
- Radiation leukemia
- Radiation related neoplasm /cancer
- Radiation syndromes
- Radiation-Induced Brachial Plexopathy
- Radiculomegaly of canine teeth congenital cataract
- Radio digito facial dysplasia
- Radio renal syndrome
- Radiophobia
- Radioulnar synostosis mental retardation hypotonia
- Radioulnar synostosis retinal pigment abnormalities
- Radio-ulnar synostosis type 1
- Radio-ulnar synostosis type 2
- Radius absent anogenital anomalies
- Raine syndrome
- Rambam Hasharon syndrome
- Rambaud Galian syndrome
- Ramer Ladda syndrome
- Ramon Syndrome
- Ramos Arroyo Clark syndrome
- Ramsay Hunt paralysis syndrome
- Rapadilino syndrome
- Rapp-Hodgkin syndrome
- Rasmussen's encephalitis
- Rasmussen Johnsen Thomsen syndrome

— Rasmussen subacute encephalitis
— Ray Peterson Scott syndrome
— Raynaud's disease/phenomenon
— Rayner Lampert Rennert syndrome
— Reactive airway disease
— Reactive arthritis
— Reactive attachment disorder of early childhood
— Reactive attachment disorder of infancy
— Reactive hypoglycemia
— Reardon Hall Slaney syndrome
— Reardon Wilson Cavanagh syndrome
— Rectal neoplasm
— Rectophobia
— Rectosigmoid neoplasm
— Recurrent laryngeal papillomas
— Recurrent peripheral facial palsy
— Recurrent respiratory papillomatosis
— Reductional transverse limb defects
— Reflex sympathetic dystrophy syndrome
— Reflux esophagitis
— Refractory anemia
— Refsum disease, infantile form
— Refsum Syndrome
— Reginato Shiapachasse syndrome
— Regional enteritis
— Reifenstein Syndrome
— Reinhardt Pfeiffer syndrome
— Reiter's Syndrome
— Renal adysplasia dominant type
— Renal agenesis meningomyelocele mullerian defect
— Renal agenesis, bilateral
— Renal agenesis
— Renal artery stenosis
— Renal calculi
— Renal caliceal diverticuli deafness
— Renal cancer
— Renal carcinoma, familial
— Renal cell carcinoma
— Renal dysplasia diffuse autosomal recessive
— Renal dysplasia diffuse cystic

— Renal dysplasia limb defects
— Renal dysplasia megalocystis sirenomelia
— Renal dysplasia mesomelia radiohumeral fusion
— Renal failure
— Renal genital middle ear anomalies
— Renal glycosuria
— Renal hepatic pancreatic dysplasia Dandy Walker cyst
— Renal hypertension
— Renal osteodystrophy
— Renal rickets
— Renal tubular acidosis progressive nerve deafness
— Renal tubular acidosis, distal, autosomal dominant
— Renal tubular acidosis, distal, autosomal recessive
— Renal tubular acidosis, distal, type 3
— Renal tubular acidosis, distal, type 4
— Renal tubular acidosis, distal
— Renal tubular acidosis
— Renal tubular transport disorders inborn
— Renier Gabreels Jasper syndrome
— Renoanogenital syndrome
— Renoprival hypertension
— Repetitive strain injury (RSI)
— Resistance to LH (luteinizing hormone)
— Resistance to thyroid stimulating hormone
— Respiratory acidosis
— Respiratory chain deficiency malformations
— Respiratory distress syndrome, Adult
— Respiratory distress syndrome, infant
— Restless legs syndrome
— Reticuloendotheliosis
— Retina disorder
— Retinal degeneration
— Retinal dysplasia X linked
— Retinal telangiectasia hypogammaglobulinemia
— Retinis pigmentosa deafness hypogenitalism
— Retinitis pigmentosa mental retardation deafness
— Retinitis pigmentosa
— Retinitis pigmentosa-deafness
— Retinoblastoma
— Retinohepatoendocrinologic syndrome

- Retinopathy anemia CNS anomalies
- Retinopathy aplastic anemia neurological abnormalities
- Retinopathy pigmentary mental retardation
- Retinopathy, arteriosclerotic
- Retinopathy, diabetic
- Retinoschisis, juvenile
- Retinoschisis, X-linked
- Retinoschisis
- Retrolental fibroplasia
- Retroperitoneal fibrosis
- Retroperitoneal liposarcoma
- Rett like syndrome
- Rett syndrome
- Revesz Debuse syndrome
- Reye's syndrome
- Reynolds Neri Hermann syndrome
- Reynolds syndrome
- Rh disease
- Rhabditida Infections
- Rhabdoid tumor
- Rhabdomyolysis
- Rhabdomyomatous dysplasia cardiopathy genital anomalies
- Rhabdomyosarcoma 1
- Rhabdomyosarcoma 2
- Rhabdomyosarcoma, alveolar
- Rhabdomyosarcoma, embryonal
- Rhabdomyosarcoma
- Rheumatic fever
- Rheumatism
- Rheumatoid arthritis
- Rheumatoid vasculitis
- Rhizomelic dysplasia type Patterson Lowry
- Rhizomelic pseudopolyarthritis
- Rhizomelic syndrome
- Rhumatoid purpura
- Rhypophobia
- Rhytiphobia
- Ribbing disease
- Richards-Rundle syndrome
- Richieri Costa Da Silva syndrome

— Richieri Costa Gorlin syndrome
— Richieri Costa Guion Almeida acrofacial dysostosis
— Richieri Costa Guion Almeida Cohen syndrome
— Richieri Costa Guion Almeida dwarfism
— Richieri Costa Guion Almeida Rodini syndrome
— Richieri Costa Montagnoli syndrome
— Richieri Costa Orquizas syndrome
— Richieri Costa Silveira Pereira syndrome
— Richieri-Costa Colletto Otto syndrome
— Richter syndrome
— Rickets
— Rickettsial disease
— Rickettsiosis
— Rieger syndrome
— Rift Valley fever
— Right atrium familial dilatation
— Right ventricle hypoplasia
— Rigid mask like face deafness polydactyly
— Rigid spine syndrome
— Riley-Day syndrome
— Ringed hair disease
— Ringworm
— Rivera Perez Salas syndrome
— Roberts Syndrome
— Robin sequence and oligodactyly
— Robinow Sorauf syndrome
— Robinow syndrome
— Robinson Miller Bensimon syndrome
— Roch-Leri mesosomatous lipomatosis
— Rocky Mountain spotted fever
— Rod myopathy
— Rodini Richieri Costa syndrome
— Rokitansky Kuster Hauser syndrome
— Rokitansky sequence
— Romano-Ward syndrome
— Romberg hemi-facial atrophy
— Rombo syndrome
— Rommen Mueller Sybert syndrome
— Rosai-Dorfman disease
— Rosenberg Chutorian syndrome

- Rosenberg Lohr syndrome
- Roseola infantum
- Rothmund-Thomson syndrome
- Rotor syndrome
- Roussy Levy hereditary areflexic dystasia
- Rowley-Rosenberg syndrome
- Roy Maroteaux Kremp syndrome
- Rozin Hertz Goodman syndrome
- Rubella virus antenatal infection
- Rubella, congenital
- Rubella
- Rubeola
- Rubinstein Taybi like syndrome
- Rubinstein-Taybi syndrome (gene promoter involvement)
- Rudd Klimek syndrome
- Rudiger syndrome
- Rumination disorder
- Rupophobia
- Rutledge Friedman Harrod syndrome
- Ruvalcaba Churesigaew Myhre syndrome
- Ruvalcaba syndrome
- Ruvalcaba-Myhre syndrome
- Ruvalcaba-Myhre-Smith syndrome (BRR)
- Ruzicka Goerz Anton syndrome

S

- Saal Bulas syndrome
- Saal Greenstein syndrome
- Sabinas brittle hair syndrome
- Saccharopinuria
- Sackey Sakati Aur syndrome
- Sacral agenesis
- Sacral defect anterior sacral meningocele
- Sacral hemangiomas multiple congenital abnormalities
- Sacral meningocele conotruncal heart defects
- Sacral plexopathy
- Sacrococcygeal dysgenesis association
- Saethre-Chotzen syndrome
- Saito Kuba Tsuruta syndrome
- Sakati syndrome

— Salcedo syndrome
— Salivary disorder
— Salivary gland disorders
— Salla disease
— Sallis Beighton syndrome
— Salmonellosis (Salmonella infections)
— Salti Salem syndrome
— Sammartino Decreccio syndrome
— Sam Spranger
— Samson Gardner syndrome
— Samson Viljoen syndrome
— Sanderson Fraser syndrome
— Sandhaus Ben Ami syndrome
— Sandhoff disease
— Sandrow Sullivan Steel syndrome
— Sanfilippo syndrome
— Santavuori disease
— Santos Mateus Leal syndrome
— SAPHO syndrome
— Sarcoidosis, pulmonary
— Sarcoidosis
— Sarcoma, Granulocytic
— Sarcosinemia
— Satoyoshi syndrome
— Saul Wilkes Stevenson syndrome
— Say Barber Hobbs syndrome
— Say Barber Miller syndrome
— Say Carpenter syndrome
— Say Field Coldwell syndrome
— Say Meyer syndrome
— Scabies
— SCAD deficiency
— Scalp defects postaxial polydactyly
— Scalp ear nipple syndrome
— Scapuloiliac dysostosis
— Scapuloperoneal myopathy
— SCARF syndrome
— Scarlet fever
— Schaap Taylor Baraitser syndrome
— Schaefer Stein Oshman syndrome

— Schamberg's disease pigmentation disorder
— Schamberg's disease
— Scheie syndrome
— Schereshevskij Turner
— Scheurermann's disease
— Schimke syndrome
— Schindler disease
— Schinzel-Giedion syndrome
— Schinzel syndrome
— Schinzel-Giedion midface retraction syndrome
— Schisis association
— Schistosomiasis
— Schizencephaly
— Schizophrenia
— Schizophrenia mental retardation deafness retinitis
— Schizophrenia, genetic types
— Schlegelberger Grote syndrome
— Schmidt syndrome
— Schmitt Gillenwater Kelly syndrome
— Schneckenbecken dysplasia
— Schofer Beetz Bohl syndrome
— Scholte Begeer Van Essen syndrome
— Schraderman's disease
— Schrander Stumpel Theunissen Hulsmans syndrome
— Schroer Hammer Mauldin syndrome
— Schwannoma, malignant
— Schwannomatosis
— Schwartz Newark syndrome
— Schwartz-Jampel syndrome
— Schwartz-lelek syndrome
— Schweitzer Kemink Malcolm syndrome
— Sciatica
— Scimitar syndrome
— Sciophobia
— Scleredema
— Scleroatonic myopathy
— Sclerocornea, Syndactyly, ambiguous genitalia
— Scleroderma
— Scleromyxedema
— Sclerosing bone dysplasia mental retardation

— Sclerosing cholangitis
— Sclerosing Lymphocytic Lobulitis
— Sclerosing Mesenteritis
— Sclerosteosis
— Sclerotylosis
— Scoleciphobia
— Scoliosis as part of NF
— Scoliosis with unilateral unsegmented bar
— Scopophobia
— SCOT deficiency
— Scotomaphobia
— Scott Bryant Graham syndrome
— Scott syndrome
— Scrapie
— Scurvy
— Sea-blue histiocytosis
— Seafood poisoning
— Seaver Cassidy syndrome
— Sebocystomatosis
— Secernentea Infections
— Seckel like syndrome Majoor Krakauer type
— Seckel like syndrome type Buebel
— Seckel syndrome 2
— Seckel syndrome
— Secondary pulmonary hypertension
— Seemanova Lesny syndrome
— Seemanova syndrome type 2
— Seghers syndrome
— Segmental neurofibromatosis
— Segmental vertebral anomalies
— Seizures benign familial neonatal recessive form
— Seizures mental retardation hair dysplasia
— Selective mutism
— Selenium poisoning
— Selenophobia
— Selig Benacerraf Greene syndrome
— Seminoma
— Semmerkrot Haraldsson Weenaes syndrome
— Sener syndrome
— Sengers Hamel Otten syndrome

- Senior syndrome
- Senior-Loken Syndrome
- Sennetsu Fever
- Sensorineural hearing loss
- Sensory neuropathy type 1
- Sensory neuropathy
- Sensory radicular neuropathy recessive form
- Senter syndrome
- Seow Najjar syndrome
- Seplophobia
- Sepsis
- Septooptic dysplasia digital anomalies
- Septo-optic dysplasia
- Sequeiros Sack syndrome
- Seres Santamaria Arimany Muniz syndrome
- Serum sickness
- Serious digitalis intoxication
- Setleis syndrome
- Severe acute respiratory syndrome (SARS)
- Severe combined immunodeficiency (SCID)
- Severe Infantile Axonal Neuropathy
- Sex Chromosome Disorders
- Sezary syndrome
- Sezary's lymphoma
- Shapiro syndrome
- Sharma Kapoor Ramji syndrome
- Sharp syndrome
- Shaver's Disease
- Sheehan syndrome
- Shigellosis
- Shingles
- Shith Filkins syndrome
- Shock
- Shokeir syndrome
- Short bowel syndrome
- Short broad great toe macrocranium
- Short chain Acyl CoA dehydrogenase deficiency
- Short limb dwarf lethal Colavita Kozlowski type
- Short limb dwarf lethal Mcalister Crane type
- Short limb dwarf oedema iris coloboma

— Short limb dwarfism Al Gazali type
— Short limbs abnormal face congenital heart disease
— Short limbs subluxed knees cleft palate
— Short QT syndrome
— Short rib syndrome Beemer type
— Short rib-polydactyly syndrome, Beermer type
— Short rib-polydactyly syndrome, Majewski type
— Short rib-polydactyly syndrome, Saldino-Noonan type
— Short rib-polydactyly syndrome, Verma-Naumoff type
— Short rib-polydactyly syndrome
— Short ribs craniosynostosis polysyndactyly
— Short stature abnormal skin pigmentation mental retardation
— Short stature Brussels type
— Short stature contractures hypotonia
— Short stature cranial hyperostosis hepatomegaly
— Short stature deafness neutrophil dysfunction
— Short stature dysmorphic face pelvic scapula dysplasia
— Short stature heart defect craniofacial anomalies
— Short stature hyperkaliemia acidosis
— Short stature locking fingers
— Short stature mental retardation eye anomalies
— Short stature mental retardation eye defects
— Short stature microcephaly heart defect
— Short stature microcephaly seizures deafness
— Short stature monodactylous ectrodactyly cleft palate
— Short stature prognathism short femoral necks
— Short stature Robin sequence cleft mandible hand anomalies clubfoot
— Short stature talipes natal teeth
— Short stature valvular heart disease
— Short stature webbed neck heart disease
— Short stature wormian bones dextrocardia
— Short syndrome
— Short tarsus absence of lower eyelashes
— Shoulder and thorax deformity congenital heart disease
— Shoulder girdle defect mental retardation familial
— Shprintzen Golberg craniosynostosis
— Shprintzen syndrome
— Shulman-Upshaw syndrome
— Shwachman syndrome

— Shwachman-Diamond syndrome
— Shwartzman phenomenon
— Shy-Drager syndrome
— Sialadenitis
— Sialidosis type 1 and 3
— Sialidosis
— Sialuria, French type
— Sickle cell anemia
— Sickle cell crisis
— Sickle cell trait
— Sideroblastic anemia, autosomal
— Siderosis
— Siegler Brewer Carey syndrome
— Silengo Lerone Pelizzo syndrome
— Silent sinus syndrome
— Silicosiderosis
— Silicosis
— Sillence syndrome
— Silver-Russell dwarfism
— Silvery hair syndrome
— Simian B virus infection
— Simosa Penchaszadeh Bustos syndrome
— Simpson-Golabi-Behmel syndrome
— Singh Chhaparwal Dhanda syndrome
— Single upper central incisor
— Single ventricular heart
— Singleton Merten syndrome
— Sinistrophobia
— Sino-auricular heart block
— Sinus cancer
— Sinus histiocytosis
— Sinus node disease and myopia
— Sipple syndrome
— Sirenomelia
— Sitophobia
— Sitosterolemia
— Situs inversus totalis with cystic dysplasia of kidneys and pancreas
— Situs inversus viscerum-cardiopathy
— Situs inversus, X linked

— Sjogren Larsson like syndrome
— Sjogren Larsson syndrome
— Sjogren's syndrome
— Skeletal dysplasia brachydactyly
— Skeletal dysplasia epilepsy short stature
— Skeletal dysplasia orofacial anomalies
— Skeletal dysplasia San diego type
— Skeletal dysplasias
— Skeleto cardiac syndrome with thrombocytopenia
— Sketetal dysplasia coarse facies mental retardation
— Skin peeling syndrome
— Slavotinek Hurst syndrome
— Sly syndrome
— Small cell lung cancer
— Small non-cleaved cell lymphoma
— Smallpox
— Smet Fabry Fryns syndrome
— Smith Fineman Myers syndrome
— Smith Martin Dodd syndrome
— Smith-Magenis Syndrome
— Sneddon Syndrome
— Sociophobia
— Soft tissue sarcoma
— Sohval Soffer syndrome
— Somatostatinoma
— Sommer Hines syndrome
— Sommer Rathbun Battles syndrome
— Sommer Young Wee Frye syndrome
— Somniphobia
— Sondheimer syndrome
— Sonoda syndrome
— Sophophobia
— Sosby syndrome
— Sotos syndrome
— Southwestern Athabaskan genetic diseases
— Sparse hair ptosis mental retardation
— Spasmodic dysphonia
— Spasmodic torticollis
— Spastic angina with healthy coronary artery
— Spastic ataxia Charlevoix-Saguenay type

— Spastic diplegia infantile type
— Spastic dysphonia
— Spastic paraparesis deafness
— Spastic paraparesis, infantile
— Spastic paraparesis
— Spastic paraplegia epilepsy mental retardation
— Spastic paraplegia facial cutaneous lesions
— Spastic paraplegia familial autosomal recessive form
— Spastic paraplegia glaucoma precocious puberty
— Spastic paraplegia mental retardation corpus callosum
— Spastic paraplegia nephritis deafness
— Spastic paraplegia neuropathy poikiloderma
— Spastic paraplegia type 1, X-linked
— Spastic paraplegia type 2, X-linked
— Spastic paraplegia type 3, dominant
— Spastic paraplegia type 4, dominant
— Spastic paraplegia type 5A, recessive
— Spastic paraplegia type 5B, recessive
— Spastic paraplegia type 6, dominant
— Spastic paraplegia, familial
— Spastic paresis glaucoma mental retardation
— Spastic quadriplegia retinitis pigmentosa mental retardation
— Spasticity mental retardation
— Spasticity multiple exostoses
— Spatic paraparesis vitiligo premature graying
— Spellacy gibbs watts syndrome
— Spermatogenesis arrest
— Spherocytosis
— Spherophakia brachymorphia syndrome
— Sphingolipidosis
— Spielmeyer-Vogt disease
— Spina bifida
— Spina bifida hypospadias
— Spinal atrophy ophthalmoplegia pyramidal syndrome
— Spinal bulbar motor neuropathy
— Spinal bulbar muscular atrophy
— Spinal cord disorder
— Spinal cord injury
— Spinal cord neoplasm
— Spinal dysostosis type Anhalt

— Spinal muscular atrophy type 1
— Spinal muscular atrophy type 2
— Spinal muscular atrophy type 3
— Spinal muscular atrophy type I with congenital bone fractures
— Spinal muscular atrophy
— Spinal shock
— Spinal stenosis
— Spine rigid cardiomyopathy
— Spinocerebellar ataxia (multiple types)
— Spinocerebellar ataxia amyotrophy deafness
— Spinocerebellar ataxia dysmorphism
— Spinocerebellar atrophy type 3
— Spinocerebellar degeneration corneal dystrophy
— Spinocerebellar degenerescence book type
— Spirochetes disease
— Spirurida Infections
— Spleen neoplasm
— Splenic agenesis syndrome
— Splenic-flexure syndrome
— Stickler syndrome, type 3
— Stickler syndrome
— Stiff man syndrome
— Stiff skin syndrome
— Still's disease
— Stimmler syndrome
— Stoelinga de koomen davis syndrome
— Stoll alembik dott syndrome
— Stoll alembik finck syndrome
— Stoll geraudel chauvin syndrome
— Stoll kieny dott syndrome
— Stoll levy francfort syndrome
— Stomach cancer, familial
— Stomach cancer
— Stomatitis
— Storage pool platelet disease
— Stormorken sjaastad langslet syndrome
— Strabismus
— Stratton garcia young syndrome
— Stratton parker syndrome
— Streeter's (Amniotic Bands)

— Streptococcus, Group B
— Strep throat
— Striatonigral degeneration infantile
— Strongyloidiasis
— Strudwick Syndrome
— Strumpell-lorrain disease
— Stuart factor deficiency, congenital
— Stuccokeratosis
— Sturge-Weber syndrome
— Stuve Wiedemann dysplasia
— Subacute cerebellar degeneration
— Subacute sclerosing leucoencephalitis
— Subacute sclerosing panencephalitis
— Subaortic stenosis short stature syndrome
— Subcortical laminar heterotopia
— Subependymal nodular heterotopia
— Subpulmonary stenosis
— Subvalvular aortic stenosis
— Succinate coenzyme Q reductase deficiency of
— Succinic acidemia lactic acidosis congenital
— Succinic acidemia
— Succinic semialdehyde dehydrogenase deficiency
— Succinyl-CoA acetoacetate transferase deficiency
— Sucrase-isomaltase deficiency
— Sudden infant death syndrome
— Sugarman syndrome
— Sulfatidosis juvenile, Austin type
— Sulfite and xanthine oxydase deficiency
— Sulfite oxidase deficiency
— Summitt syndrome
— Super mesenteric artery syndrome
— Supranuclear ocular palsy
— Supraumbilical midabdominal raphe and facial cavernous hemangiomas
— Suriphobia
— Susac syndrome
— Sutherland Haan syndrome
— Sutton disease II
— Sutton's Disease II
— Sweeley-Klionsky disease

— Sweet syndrome
— Swimmer's ear
— Swyer James and McLeod Syndrome
— Swyer syndrome
— Sybert Smith syndrome
— Sydenham's chorea
— Symmetrical thalamic calcifications
— Symphalangism brachydactyly craniosynostosis
— Symphalangism brachydactyly
— Symphalangism Cushing type
— Symphalangism distal
— Symphalangism familial proximal
— Symphalangism short stature accessory testis
— Symphalangism with multiple anomalies of hands and feet
— Symphalangism, distal, with microdontia, dental pulp stones, and narrowed zygomatic arch
— Syncamptodactyly scoliosis
— Syncopal paroxysmal tachycardia
— Syncopal tachyarythmia
— Syncope
— Syndactyly between 4 and 5
— Syndactyly cataract mental retardation
— Syndactyly Cenani Lenz type
— Syndactyly ectodermal dysplasia cleft lip palate hand foot
— Syndactyly type 1 microcephaly mental retardation
— Syndactyly type 2
— Syndactyly type 3
— Syndactyly type 5
— Syndactyly
— Syndactyly-polydactyly-ear lobe syndrome
— Syndrome of inappropraite antidiuretic hormone
— Syndrome X
— Syngnathia cleft palate
— Syngnathia multiple anomalies
— Synostosis of talus and calcaneus short stature
— Synovial cancer
— Synovial osteochondromatosis
— Synovial sarcoma
— Synovialosarcoma
— Synovitis acne pustulosis hyperostosis osteitis

— Synovitis granulomatous uveitis cranial neuropathi
— Synovitis
— Synpolydactyly
— Syphilis embryopathy
— Syphilis
— Syringobulbia
— Syringocystadenoma papilliferum
— Syringomas
— Syringomas natal teeth oligodontia
— Syringomelia hyperkeratosis
— Syringomyelia
— Systemic arterio-veinous fistula
— Systemic carnitine deficiency
— Systemic lupus erythematosus
— Systemic mastocytosis
— Systemic necrotizing angeitis
— Systemic sclerosis

T

— T cell immunodeficiency primary
— Tabatznik syndrome
— Tachycardia
— Taeniasis
— Takayasu arteritis
— Talipes equinovarus
— Tamari Goodman syndrome
— Tang Hsi Ryu syndrome
— Tangier disease
— TAR syndrome
— Tardive dyskinesia
— Tarsal tunnel syndrome
— Taste disorder
— TAU syndrome
— Taurodontia absent teeth sparse hair
— Taurodontism
— Tay syndrome ichthyosis
— Taybi Linder syndrome
— Taybi syndrome
— Tay-Sachs disease
— T-cell lymphoma

— Teebi Kaurah syndrome
— Teebi Naguib Alawadi syndrome
— Teebi Shaltout syndrome
— Teebi syndrome
— Teeth noneruption of with maxillary hypoplasia and genu valgum
— Tel Hashomer camptodactyly syndrome
— Telangiectasia ataxia variant V1
— Telangiectasia, hereditary hemorrhagic
— Telangiectasia
— Telecanthus hypertelorism pes cavus
— Telecanthus with associated abnormalities
— Telencephalic leukoencephalopathy
— Telfer Sugar Jaeger syndrome
— Temporal epilepsy, familial
— Temporomandibular ankylosis
— Temporomandibular joint dysfunction (TMJ)
— Temtamy Shalash syndrome
— TEN
— Ter Haar Hamel Hendricks syndrome
— Ter Haar syndrome
— Teratocarcinosarcoma
— Teratoma
— Teratophobia
— Testes neoplasm
— Testotoxicosis
— Tetanophobia
— Tetanus
— Tethered spinal cord disease
— Tetraamelia ectodermal dysplasia
— Tetraamelia multiple malformations
— Tetraamelia pulmonary hypoplasia
— Tetraamelia-syrinx
— Tetrahydrobiopterin deficiencies
— Tetraploidy
— Tetrasomy X
— Thakker Donnai syndrome
— Thalamic degeneration symmetrical infantile
— Thalamic degenerescence infantile
— Thalamic syndrome
— Thalassemia major

— Thalassemia minor
— Thalassemia
— Thanatophobia
— Thanatophoric dysplasia cloverleaf skull
— Thanatophoric dysplasia Glasgow variant
— Thanos Stewart Zonana syndrome
— Theodor Hertz Goodman syndrome
— Thiele syndrome
— Thiemann epiphyseal disease
— Thies Reis syndrome
— Thin ribs tubular bones dysmorphism
— Thiolase deficiency
— Thiopurine S methyltranferase deficiency
— Thomas Jewett Raines syndrome
— Thomas syndrome
— Thombocytopenia X linked
— Thompson Baraitser syndrome
— Thong Douglas Ferrante syndrome
— Thoracic celosomia
— Thoracic dysplasia hydrocephalus syndrome
— Thoracic outlet syndrome
— Thoraco abdominal enteric duplication
— Thoraco limb dysplasia Rivera type
— Thoracolaryngopelvic dysplasia
— Thoracopelvic dysostosis
— Thost-Unna palmoplantar keratoderma
— Thrombasthenia
— Thrombocytopathy asplenia miosis
— Thrombocytopathy
— Thrombocytopenia cerebellar hypoplasia short stature
— Thrombocytopenia chromosome breakage
— Thrombocytopenia multiple congenital anomaly
— Thrombocytopenia purpura
— Thrombocytopenia Robin sequence
— Thrombocytopenia
— Thrombocytopenic purpura, autoimmune
— Thrombocytosis
— Thrombomodulin anomalies, familial
— Thrombotic microangiopathy, familial
— Thrush

— Thumb absence hypoplastic halluces
— Thumb absent short stature immune deficiency
— Thumb deformity, alopecia, pigmentation anomaly
— Thumb deformity
— Thumb stiff brachydactyly mental retardation
— Thymic carcinoma
— Thymic epithelial tumor
— Thymic renal anal lung dysplasia
— Thymoma
— Thymus neoplasm
— Thyrocerebrorenal syndrome
— Thyroglossal tract cyst
— Thyroid agenesis
— Thyroid cancer
— Thyroid carcinoma, follicular
— Thyroid carcinoma, papillary (TPC)
— Thyroid hormone plasma membrane transport defect
— Thyroid, renal and digital anomalies
— Tibia absent polydactyly arachnoid cyst
— Tibiae bowed radial anomalies osteopenia fracture
— Tibial aplasia ectrodactyly hydrocephalus
— Tibial aplasia ectrodactyly
— Tibial hemimelia cleft lip palate
— Tick paralysis
— Tick-borne encephalitis
— Tièche-Jadassohn nevus
— Tietz syndrome
— Tinnitus
— T-Lymphocytopenia
— Todd's paralysis
— Togaviridae disease
— Tollner Horst Manzke syndrome
— Tolosa-Hunt syndrome
— Toluene antenatal infection
— Tomaculous neuropathy
— Tome Brune Fardeau syndrome
— Tongue neoplasm
— Toni Debre Fanconi maladie
— Toni-Fanconi syndrome
— Topophobia

— TORCH syndrome
— Toriello Carey syndrome
— Toriello Lacassie Droste syndrome
— Toriello syndrome
— Transverse limb deficiency hemangioma
— Transverse myelitis
— TRAPS (TNF-receptor-associated periodic syndrome)
— Traumatophobia
— Treacher Collins syndrome
— Treft Sanborn Carey syndrome
— Tremophobia
— Tremor hereditary essential
— Treponema infection
— Trevor disease
— Triatrial heart
— Trichinellosis
— Trichinosis
— Tricho dento osseous syndrome type 1
— Tricho odonto onycho dermal syndrome
— Tricho odonto onychodysplasia syndactyly dominant type
— Tricho onychic dysplasia
— Tricho onycho hypohidrotic dysplasia
— Tricho retino dento digital syndrome
— Trichodental syndrome
— Tricho-dento-osseous syndrome
— Trichodermodysplasia dental alterations
— Trichodysplasia xeroderma
— Trichoepithelioma multiple familial
— Trichofolliculloma
— Tricho-hepato-enteric syndrome
— Trichomalacia
— Trichomegaly cataract hereditary spherocytosis
— Trichomegaly retina pigmentary degeneration dwarfi
— Trichomoniasis
— Trichoodontoonychial dysplasia
— Trichopathophobia
— Trichorhinophalangeal syndrome type I
— Trichorhinophalangeal syndrome type II
— Trichorhinophalangeal syndrome type III
— Trichostasis spinulosa

— Trichothiodystrophy sun sensitivity
— Trichothiodystrophy
— Trichotillomania
— Tricuspid atresia
— Tricuspid dysplasia
— Trigeminal neuralgia
— Trigger thumb
— Trigonocephaly bifid nose acral anomalies
— Trigonocephaly broad thumbs
— Trigonocephaly ptosis coloboma
— Trigonocephaly ptosis mental retardation
— Trigonomacrocephaly tibial defect polydactyly
— Trihydroxycholestanoylcoa oxidase isolated deficiency
— Trimethadione antenatal infection
— Trimethylaminuria
— Triopia
— Triose phosphate-isomerase deficiency
— Triphalangeal thumb non opposable
— Triphalangeal thumb polysyndactyly syndrome
— Triphalangeal thumbs brachyectrodactyly
— Triple A syndrome
— Triplo X Syndrome
— Triploid Syndrome
— Triploidy
— Trypanosomiasis, west African
— Tsao Ellingson syndrome
— Tsukahara Azuno Kajii syndrome
— Tsukahara Kajii syndrome
— Tsukuhara syndrome
— Tuberculophobia
— Tuberculosis, pulmonary
— Tuberculosis
— Tuberculous meningitis
— Tuberculous uveitis
— Tuberous Sclerosis, type 1
— Tuberous Sclerosis, type 2
— Tuberous Sclerosis
— Tucker syndrome
— Tuffli Laxova syndrome
— Tufted angioma

— Tularemia
— Tungiasis
— Tunglang Savage Bellman syndrome
— Turcot syndrome
— Turner Kieser syndrome
— Turner Morgani Albright
— Turner-like syndrome
— Turner's syndrome
— Tutuncuoglu syndrome
— Twin twin transfusion syndrome
— Typhoid
— Typhus
— Tyrosinemia
— Tyrosine-oxidase temporary deficiency

U

— UDP-galactose-4-epimerase deficiency
— Uhl anomaly
— Ulbright Hodes syndrome
— Ulcerative colitis
— Ulerythema ophryogenesis
— Ulna and fibula absence with severe limb deficit
— Ulna hypoplasia mental retardation
— Ulna metaphyseal dysplasia syndrome
— Ulnar hypoplasia lobster claw deformity of feet
— Umbilical cord ulceration intestinal atresia
— Uniparental disomy
— Unna-Politzer nevus
— Unna's seborrhoeic eczema
— Upington disease
— Upper limb defect eye and ear abnormalities
— Upton Young syndrome
— Urachal cancer
— Urachal cyst
— Uramoron syndrome
— Urban Rogers Meyer syndrome
— Urban Schosser Spohn syndrome
— Urea cycle enzymopathies
— Uremia
— Urethral obstruction sequence

— Uridine monophosphate synthetase deficiency
— Urinary calculi
— Urinary tract neoplasm
— Urioste Martinez Frias syndrome
— Urocanase deficiency
— Urogenital adysplasia
— Urophathy distal obstructive polydactyly
— Urticaria pigmentosa
— Urticaria
— Urticaria-deafness-amyloidosis
— Usher syndrome, type 1C
— Usher syndrome, type 1D
— Usher syndrome, type 1E
— Usher syndrome, type 2A
— Usher syndrome, type 2B
— Usher syndrome, type 2C
— Usher syndrome, type 3
— Usher syndrome, type IA
— Usher syndrome, type IB
— Usher syndrome
— Uveal diseases
— Uveitis, anterior
— Uveitis, posterior
— Uveitis

V

— Vaccinophobia
— VACTERL association with hydrocephaly, X linked
— VACTERL association
— VACTERL hydrocephaly
— Vacuolar myopathy
— Vagina absence of
— Vaginismus
— Vagneur Triolle Ripert syndrome
— Valinemia
— Valproic acid antenatal infection
— Vascular malposition
— Vascular purpura
— Vasculitis
— Vasculitis hypersensitivity

— Vasculitis, cutaneous necrotizing
— Vasopressin-resistant diabetes insipidus
— Vasovagal syncope
— Vasquez Hurst Sotos syndrome
— VATER association
— Vein of Galen aneurysmal malformations (VGAM)
— Vein of Galen aneurysmal dilatation (VGAD)
— Velocardiofacial syndrome
— Velofacioskeletal syndrome
— Velopharyngeal incompetence
— Venencie Powell Winkelmann syndrome
— Ventricular extrasystoles perodactyly Robin sequence
— Ventricular familial preexcitation syndrome
— Ventricular fibrillation, idiopathic
— Ventricular septal defect
— Ventriculo-arterial discordance, isolated
— Ventruto Digirolamo Festa syndrome
— Verloes Bourguignon syndrome
— Verloes David syndrome
— Verloes Gillerot Fryns syndrome
— Verloes Van Maldergem Marneffe syndrome
— Verloove Vanhorick Brubakk syndrome
— Verminiphobia
— Vernal keratoconjunctivitis
— Verrucous nevus acanthokeratolytic
— Verrucous nevus
— Vertebral body fusion overgrowth
— Vertebral fusion posterior lumbosacral blepharoptosis
— Vertical talus
— Vestibulocochlear dysfunction progressive familial
— Viljoen Kallis Voges syndrome
— Viljoen Smart syndrome
— Viljoen Winship syndrome
— Vipoma
— Viral hemorrhagic fever
— Virilism
— Virilizing ovarian tumor
— Virus associated hemophagocytic syndrome
— Visceral myopathy familial external ophthalmoplegia
— Vitamin A embryopathy

— Vitamin B 6 Deficiency
— Vitamin B12 Deficiency
— Vitamin B12 responsive methylmalonic acidemia, cbl A
— Vitamin B12 responsive methylmalonicaciduria
— Vitamin D resistant rickets
— Vitamin E deficiency
— Vitamin E familial isolated, deficiency of
— Vitiligo mental retardation facial dysmorphism uremia
— Vitiligo psychomotor retardation cleft palate facial dysmorphism
— Vitiligo
— Vitreoretinal degeneration
— Vitreoretinochoroidopathy dominant
— VKH
— VLCAD deficiency
— Vocal cord dysfunction familial
— Von Gierke disease
— Von Hippel-Lindau disease
— Von Recklinghausen disease
— Von Voss Cherstvoy syndrome
— Von Willebrand disease
— Vulvodynia
— Vulvovaginitis

W

— W syndrome
— Waaler Aarskog syndrome
— Waardenburg syndrome type 1
— Waardenburg syndrome type 2
— Waardenburg syndrome type 2A
— Waardenburg syndrome type 2B
— Waardenburg syndrome type 3
— Waardenburg syndrome, type 4
— Waardenburg syndrome
— Waardenburg type Pierpont
— Wagner's disease
— Wagner-Stickler syndrome
— WAGR syndrome
— Walbaum Titran Durieux Crepin syndrome
— Waldenstrom macroglobulinemia
— Waldmann disease

— Walker Dyson syndrome
— Wallerian degeneration
— Wallis Zieff Goldblatt syndrome
— Wandering spleen
— Warburg Sjo Fledelius syndrome
— Warburg Thomsen syndrome
— Warburton Anyane Yeboa syndrome
— Wells Jankovic syndrome
— Wells syndrome
— Werdnig-Hoffmann disease
— Wheat Hypersensitivity
— Whipple disease
— Whitaker syndrome
— White matter hypoplasia corpus callosum agenesia mental retardation
— White sponge nevus of cannon
— Whooping cough (Pertussis)
— Whyte Murphy syndrome
— Wieacker syndrome
— Williams syndrome
— Wilms tumor and pseudohermaphroditism
— Wilms tumor radial bilateral aplasia
— Wright Dick syndrome
— Wrinkly skin syndrome
— Writer's cramp
— Wt limb blood syndrome
— Wyburn-Mason's syndrome

X

— X chromosome, duplication Xq13 1 q21 1
— X chromosome, monosomy Xp22 pter
— X chromosome, monosomy Xq28
— X chromosome, trisomy Xp3
— X chromosome, trisomy Xpter Xq13
— X chromosome, trisomy Xq
— X chromosome, trisomy Xq25
— X fragile site folic acid type
— Xanthic urolithiasis
— Xanthine oxydase deficiency
— Xanthinuria

— Xanthomatosis cerebrotendinous
— Xanthophobia
— Xenoglossophobia
— Xenophobia
— Xerocytosis, hereditary
— Xeroderma pigmentosum, type 1
— Xeroderma pigmentosum, type 2
— Xeroderma pigmentosum, type 3
— Xeroderma pigmentosum, type 5
— Xeroderma pigmentosum, type 6
— Xeroderma pigmentosum, type 7
— Xeroderma pigmentosum, variant type
— Xeroderma pigmentosum
— Xeroderma talipes enamel defects
— Xerophobia
— Xk aprosencephaly
— X-linked adrenal hypoplasia congenita
— X-linked alpha thalassemia mental retardation syndrome (ATR-X)
— X-linked dominant
— X-linked ichthyosis
— X-linked juvenile retinoschisis
— X-linked juvenile retinoschisis
— X-linked lymphoproliferative syndrome
— X-linked mental retardation and macro-orchidism
— X-linked mental retardation associated with marXq2
— X-linked mental retardation Brooks type
— X-linked mental retardation craniofacial abnormal microcephaly club
— X-linked mental retardation De silva type
— X-linked mental retardation Hamel type
— X-linked mental retardation type Gustavson
— X-linked mental retardation type Martinez
— X-linked mental retardation type Raynaud
— X-linked mental retardation type Schutz
— X-linked mental retardation type Snyder
— X-linked mental retardation type Wittner
— X-linked mental retardation-hypotonia
— X-linked severe combined immunodeficiency
— X-linked trait

— XX male syndrome
— XY Female
— XY gonadal agenesis syndrome
— Xylophobia

Y

— Y chromosome deletions
— Yaws
— Yellow fever
— Yellow nail syndrome
— Yersinia pestis
— Yersiniosis
— Yim Ebbin syndrome
— Yolk sac tumor
— Yorifuji Okuno syndrome
— Yoshimura-Takeshita syndrome
— Young Hugues syndrome
— Young Maders syndrome
— Young Mc keever Squier syndrome
— Young Simpson syndrome
— Young Syndrome
— Yunis Varon syndrome
— Yusho Disease

Z

— Zadik Barak Levin syndrome
— ZAP70 deficiency
— Zazam Sheriff Phillips syndrome
— Zellweger syndrome
— Zimmerman Laband syndrome
— Zlotogora syndrome
— Zollinger-Ellison syndrome
— Zonular cataract and nystagmus
— Zori Stalker Williams syndrome
— Zunich-Kaye syndrome
— Zuska's Disease

Bibliography

Battles JB, Kaplan HS, Van der Schaaf TW, Shea CE. The attributes of medical event-reporting systems: experience with a prototype medical event-reporting system for transfusion medicine. *Arch Pathol Lab Med* 1998; 122:231-238.

Berman S. Identifying and addressing sentinel events: an Interview with Richard Croteau. *Jt Comm J Qual Improv* 1998; 24:426-434.

Bhasale A. The wrong diagnosis: identifying causes of potentially adverse events in general practice using incident monitoring. *Fam Pract* 1998; 15:308-318.

Caplan RA, Posner KL, Cheney FW. Effect of outcome on physician judgments of appropriateness of care. *JAMA* 1991; 265:1957-1960.

Eagle CJ, Davies JM, Reason J. Accident analysis of large-scale technological disasters applied to an anaesthetic complication. *Can J Anaesth* 1992; 39:118-122.

Fernandes CM, Walker R, Price A, Marsden J, Haley L. Root cause analysis of laboratory delays to an emergency department. *J Emerg Med* 1997; 15:735-739.

Giacomini MK, Cook DJ. Users' guides to the medical literature: XXIII. Qualitative research in health care A. Are the results of the study valid? Evidence-Based Medicine Working Group. *JAMA* 2000; 284:357-362.

Joint Commission on the Accreditation of Healthcare Organisations. Sentinel event policy and procedures.

Available at: http://www.JCAHO.org/sentinel/se_pp.html. Accessed May 30, 2001.

Kaplan HS, Battles JB, Van der Schaaf TW, Shea CE, Mercer SQ. Identification and classification of the causes of events in transfusion medicine. *Transfusion* 1998; 38:1071-1081.

Sazama K. Reports of 355 transfusion-associated deaths: 1976 through 1985. *Transfusion* 1990; 30:583-590.

Troidl H. Disasters of endoscopic surgery and how to avoid them: error analysis. *World J Surg* 1999; 23:846-855.

Van der Schaaf T. Near miss reporting in the Chemical Process Industry [Doctoral thesis]. Eindhoven, The Netherlands: Eindhoven University of Technology. 1992.

Vincent C, Ennis M, Audley RJ. *Medical accidents*. Oxford; New York: Oxford University Press. 1993.

Index

A

ABCD syndrome, 170
Abdominal neoplasms, 170
Acanthocytosis, 170
Accessory pancreas, 171
Achromatopsia, 171
Ackerman syndrome, 171
Acquired syphilis, 171
Acrodysostosis, 172
Acromicric dysplasia, 172
Adenocarcinoid tumor, 174
Advanced life support, 27
AIIMS, 77
Allergic angiitis, 175
Amblyopia, 177
Ambulance attendant, 28
Ambulance, 27
Ambulatory surgical care, 6
Amenorrhea, 177
American Red Cross, 39
Anaesthesiology, 75
Anesthesia Services, 52
Appropriate hospital fees, 6
Argyria, 181
Autonomous facilities, 3

B

BAER, 183
Ballard syndrome, 183
Basic life support, 28
Basic Life Support, 49
Berylliosis, 185
Biochemistry, 56
Blepharophimosis, 186
Blood bank, 75
Blood counts, 60
BLS, 28
BOD syndrome, 187
Boder syndrome, 187
Borreliosis, 187
Botulism, 187
Bridgeport Hospital, 24

C

CACH syndrome, 190
Calciphylaxis, 190
Callus disease, 191
Capos syndrome, 191
Cardiac malformation, 192
Care after Discharge, 20
Carney syndrome, 193

CEMIC, 88
Central Pathology Laboratory, 61
Ceraunophobia, 195
Chikungunya, 198
Chorea, 199
Clinical Pharmacology, 75
Critical Illness, 21
CRNA, 53

D

Dementophobia, 207
DEMSOC, 46, 50
Disaster planning, 44
DOH, 2, 4, 6, 10, 13
  botika, 7
  budget, 2
  indigency funds, 8
  priorities, 7
Domiciliary care, 6
DPH, 22, 23, 26

E

EAF, 213
Early defibrillation,
  provider, 29
  service, 29
Elephantiasis, 215
Emergency medical,
  dispatchers, 38
  Services, 21, 36, 46
    System, 22, 29
Emergency medical technician, 29
EMS, 21, 25, 35, 44
  delivery system, 25
  providers, 50
  system, 22, 44
EMSS, 29
EMT, 29
Endocrinology, 75
Expensive component, 1
External funding sources, 7

F

Fascioliasis, 219
FLENI, 88
Fortis Health Care Limited, 77
FRAXD, 222

G

Gastroenterology, 75
General Hospital Laboratory, 58
Genu varum, 225
Ghosal syndrome, 225
Glioblastoma, 226
Glucagonoma, 227

H

Hallux valgus, 230
Hartford Hospital, 24
Health,
  facility development, 9
  insurance coverage, 2
  insurance system, 7
  planning agencies, 30
  services, 1

Hearing impairment, 231
Helminthiasis, 60
Histidinemia, 235
Hospital,
 administration, 38
 authority, 69
 development plans, 3
 emergency departments, 24
 Information Systems, 13
Hurler syndrome, 237

I

Integrated Hospital Information System, 8
International Classification of Diseases, 73
Irrational delivery, 2

J

Jejunal atresia, 246
Juvenile gout, 247

K

Kabuki syndrome, 247
Kaolin pneumoconiosis, 247
Keratoconus, 248
Kernicterus, 248
Klumpke paralysis, 249
Kostmann syndrome, 249
Kyphosis, 250

L

Laboratory,
 Informatics, 58
 information system, 58
Labrador lung, 250
Lafora disease, 250
Lanier Health Services, 85
Laryngocele, 251
Laryngomalacia, 251
Leigh disease, 252
Leprosy, 252
Leucinosis, 253
Leukoplakia, 253
LGCR, 253
LGS, 253
LGU, 12, 13
Licensed practical nurses, 51
Linonophobia, 254
Liposarcoma, 254
Listeriosis, 254
Local,
 Fire Department, 23
 Health Executives, 10
 health system, 2
Logic syndrome, 255
Lowry syndrome, 255
LSA, 255
Luzon, 4
Lyme disease, 256
Lymphedema, 256
Lymphoma, 257

M

Maffucci syndrome, 258
Malonic aciduria, 259
MAMC, 77
Mass syndrome, 260
Max Hospital, 77

Medical,
Control, 30
Laboratory, 56
Park Hospital, 87
Technology, 70
Megaduodenum, 261
Meningioma, 262
Metabolic acidosis, 264
Michels syndrome, 265
Microbiology, 76
Mindanao, 4
Mobius syndrome, 267
Modi Hospital, 77
Monilethrix, 268
Mullerian agenesis, 269
Myasthenia gravis, 270
Myelinopathies, 270
Myelitis, 270
Myiasis, 271
Myoclonus, 271

N

National health budget, 1
National hospitals, 5
Negative budget, 5
Nelson syndrome, 273
Neopharmaphobia, 273
Nephrology, 76
Neurasthenia, 274
Neurofibromatosis, 274
Neurosurgery, 76
Nevo syndrome, 275
Norrie disease, 276
Nuclear Medicine Services, 54
NZEF, 65

O

Obesophobia, 276
Occupational Therapy, 76
Ockelbo disease, 276
Oculo tricho dysplasia, 277
Oculodentodigital syndrome, 277
OEMS, 23
Oikophobia, 278
Oligophernia, 278
Olmsted syndrome, 278
Ombrophobia, 278
Onchocerciasis, 278
Oncology centers, 4
Oneirophobia, 279
Opitz syndrome, 279
Optic atrophy, 279
Optic neuritis, 279
Optional Hospital, Services, 52
Oral surgeon, 53
Ornithinemia, 280
Oslam syndrome, 280
Osmed Syndrome, 280
Osteoarthritis, 280
Overutilized medical facilities, 5

P

Pachygyria, 282
Palsy cerebral, 282
Panic attacks, 18
Panophobia, 283
Paraganglioma, 283
Paraplegia, 283
Pediatric centers, 4
Pediatric Surgery, 76

Peripheral neuropathy, 14
Pharmacology, 76
Philippine Heart Center, 4
Pinnacle Pointe Hospital, 87
Potential hospital patients, 7
Practicing trauma surgeons, 38
Presbycusis, 291
Providence Hospital, 85
Public health programmes, 7
Public safety,
  agencies, 42
  personnel, 30
Puncture fluids, 60
Pyrophobia, 294

Q

Qualified anesthesiologist, 53
Qualified registered nurses, 51
Quebec platelet disorder, 295

R

Rabies, 295
Radiophobia, 295, 296
Recurrent nightmares, 18
Reflux esophagitis, 296
Regional hospitals, 5
Relapsing fever, 60
Renal,
  calculi, 296
  osteodystrophy, 297
Renoprival hypertension, 297
Retina disorder, 297
Reynolds syndrome, 298
Rheumatism, 298
Rhypophobia, 298
Rhytiphobia, 298
Richter syndrome, 299
Ringworm, 299
Robinow syndrome, 299
Rod myopathy, 299
Ruvalcaba syndrome, 300

S

Sacral agenesis, 300
SAED, 29, 46
Sakati syndrome, 300
Salla disease, 301
Sam Spranger, 301
Sample Processing, 57
SAPHO, 301
Scabies, 301
SCAD deficiency, 301
Schimke syndrome, 302
Schistosomiasis, 302
Schizencephaly, 302
Sciatica, 302
Scimitar syndrome, 302
Scleredema, 302
Scleroderma, 302
Sclerosteosis, 303
Scotomaphobia, 303
Sergeant technician, 65
Sialidosis, 306
Sinus cancer, 306
Sitosterolemia, 306
Smallpox, 307
Social isolation, 19
Sophophobia, 307

Spastic paraparesis, 308
Specialized Health Care, 4
Specialty care unit, 31, 42
Spherocytosis, 308
Spinal,
  shock, 309
  stenosis, 309
Stamford Hospital, 24
State Fire School, 38
Stuccokeratosis, 310
Surgical privileges, 51
Suriphobia, 310

T

Thomas syndrome, 314
Throat swabs, 60
Thymic carcinoma, 315
Thyroid agenesis, 315
Tinnitus, 315
Toxicology centers, 4
Trauma,
  Care System, 30
  Facility, 31
  Patient, 32
  rehabilitation professionals, 37
  Systems Committee, 33
Treatment protocols, 32
Trichinosis, 316
Typhoid fever, 62
Typhus fever, 60
Tyrosinemia, 318

U

UAB Hospital, 85
UAMS, 88
Undulant fever, 60
Uniparental disomy, 318
Upington disease, 318
Urachal cyst, 318
Uremia, 318
Urology, 76
Urticaria, 319
Usher syndrome, 319

V

Vaginismus, 319
Valinemia, 319
Vardaan Hospital, 78
Vasant Lok Hospital, 78
Venereal disease, 60
Verminiphobia, 320
Vipoma, 320
Virilism, 320
Visayas, 4
Vitiligo, 321
Volunteer Ambulance Company, 23

W

Waardenburg syndrome, 321
Waterbury Hospital, 24
Wilmington Medical Center, 39
Wound infections, 60
Wrangell Medical Center, 86

Y

Yersiniosis, 324
Yusho Disease, 324